Wolfgang Wirth

Healing with Aloe

Tissue Therapy – Aloe Therapy – Agave Healing System
The Turning Point for Many Ailments

PUBLISHING HOUSE WILHELM ENNSTHALER, STEYR

I would like to give special thanks to Mr. MICHAEL GARTZ
for his advice and co-operation.

Wolfgang Wirth

1st english edition 1986

ISBN 3 85068 213 7

TABLE OF CONTENTS

INTRODUCTION

In this publication, three new systems of healing, i. e. therapy procedures, will be introduced which are unknown in the Western industrial nations, but which have already proved to be so successful in other countries that they have been integrated into academic medicine. Perhaps it seems strange that such therapies have not yet been made available to us as patients and that their method of application has not been taught to us by academic medicine. The reason is that the positive results of these therapies are known »only« through practical experience; however, the scientific proof of the corresponding effect mechanism according to the criteria in this country is missing. This proof has now been established through the tracking down of »depots« of the biogenic stimulators. Herewith the three new therapy systems that serve to convert cellulose and which contain a broad spectrum of biological healing properties can finally be introduced on a broad scale.

I am referring to the tissue therapy, the aloe therapy, as well as the agave-cure complex. Many patients who previously could not be helped are justified in renewing their hope! When one considers that, for example, the aloe therapy improves vision and stabilizes this improvement, heals many different eye diseases, that the tormenting suffering of those afflicted with bronchial asthma can be cured or considerably relieved, that all diseases involving defects of the immune system such as cancer, multiple sclerosis or the new plague, AIDS, can be positively influenced when the new therapy is put into practice, or that the quality of life for older people and their ability to work can be maintained and increased, then it is not presumptious to speak of a turning point in biological medicine.

It does not seem to be a coincidence that, precisely in our age of radiation injuries, an active agent from the aloe should be discovered which, for the first time, affords protection against such injuries, and that healing has been achieved where burns or malignant abscesses caused by radiotherapy were present.

The whole X-ray-therapy system has herewith been given a protective and preventive measure of the first order.

For this reason, this publication belongs not only in the hands of the millions afflicted will illness, but also in those of doctors and non-medical practitioners, researchers, pharmacists, health insurance companies, hospitals and sanatoriums, those working for the World Health Organization, missions and, last but not least, the politicians responsible for our health.

Therefore, besides the popular presentation of the new healing systems and the successful treatments so far, a scientific report has also been included to make it possible for the expert reader to follow the indication claims and the working mechanism of the therapies scientifically. Those who are concerned as patients themselves will be able to look up the most effective method of application under the individually listed aspects of the case.

Above all, it will be proven to sceptical persons why the effects spectrum of this method of healing is so uncommonly wide. They will see that the active agents that have been discovered somehow correspond materially to substances in the organism; they compensate its deficiency. Research has herewith come upon elements that, in a way of speaking, constitute an alternative household for the organism, and these shall be made available to everyone through the presentation of the therapies. The sceptical doctor is invited to put the therapies, as described here, to the test. He will quickly be convinced that a remedy has been placed into his hands, which will enable him to heal serious diseases without side-effects and without counterindications; even in the absence of a definite cure, the general condition of the patient will in any case be improved.

I would like to point out one risk factor: the aloe-injection therapy should not be administered to pregnant women, because larger doses of aloe cause a congestion of blood in the pelvis.

The doses are administered by injection. This should not disturb the patient. The injections are subcutaneous, i. e. injected under the skin, and not intravenous or intramuscular, and they are completely harmless. Injections have undergone such improvements since diabetics have been using them in large quantities, that an injection with is very fine needle can hardly be felt. The author of this publication explicitly recommends the injections used by diabetics (0.5 or 1 ml, depending on therapy instructions), which are available in pharmacies.

To make it possible for everyone, the layman as well as the professionally trained person, to carry out the new biological healing system down the smallest detail, nothing will be concealed; the principle of the biogenic stimulators as well as complete prescriptions will be fully disclosed. This too is unique and intentional, as is the honesty of this publication, which propagates new biological healing systems on the basis of verifiable experience, and consequently it does not have to shun any debate with academic medicine or chemotherapy.

WOLFGANG WIRTH

IMPORTANT DIRECTIONS

Aloe in all forms of administration can be obtained without a prescription in West Germany as well as in Switzerland; in Austria amounts up to 50 mg per dose are prescription-free; anything above this amount can be had only with a prescription. Homeopathic aloe units are prescription-free in Austria only from D 4 on. Emulsions can be obtained here too without a prescription.

SPECIAL DIRECTIONS

Children should not be treated with aloe-extract injections unless they are 5 years of age or older. Treatment should be carried out by a doctor.

Although a diagnosis always belongs in the hands of a doctor, or a non-medicinal practitioner, as far as he is entitled to administer the treatment, grown-up patients can treat themselves similar to the procedure of the diabetic with the insulin injection, preferably under guidance (doctor, non-medical practitioner, medical-technical assistant, nurse) – following exactly the recommendations of this publication, or when under the care of a doctor or non-practitioner, following his instructions only.

Under the descriptions of the individual diseases, the reader will find a recommendation as to when the injections are to be administered.

Wherever this reference is missing, the injections should be given in the morning hours. In case this is inconvenient, any other time of day is possible; however, after each injection, a period of rest of about 15 minutes should be observed. Since some patients may experience a slight rise in blood pressure, these people should not receive the injections before going to sleep, unless individual therapies prescribe the opposite treatment expressly. The aloe compounds recommended in this publication must be designated as **»biostimulated«,** because the products without this designation are used as laxatives.

The injection is called ALOE D 2 - biostimulated, or ALOGEN according to Wolfgang Wirth MDH.

Further inquiries of any kind concerning the contents of this publication should not be addressed to the publishing house, but to the following address. (Please enclose pre-paid, self-addressed return envelope.)

Arbeitsgemeinschaft Grundlagenforschung für biologische Medizin
Postfach 61 0 220
D-1000 Berlin 61

A PLANT CONCEALS A SECRET

Pharmacy is not unfamiliar with the aloe, the ornamental plant with the melodious name. Various products made from it which can be used in different ways are known as laxatives. *Abführmittel*

In fact one can say that it is one of the most effective laxatives. Nevertheless, the plant conceals a secret that has now been deciphered for the benefit of health.

It comes as no great surprise that the aloe contains more healing properties than just that of a laxative. Generations of us have called the aloe, which could be found on almost every flower shelf, the »FIRST-AID« plant. Why? For cuts, an aloe leaf was broken off the bottom part of the plant and the viscid juice was applied to the wound with the result that the wound immediately closed. The blood-staunching, astringent qualities of aloe juice should long ago have induced researchers to take a closer look at the active agents contained in the aloe plant in order to make them available to mankind. This has been done just recently after Professor Vladimir Filatow*, a famous Russian oculist, made an important beginning for research by being the first to gain medical experience in applying the healing properties of this Biblical plant with enduring success. »Active agents of an unknown nature« is what Prof. Filatow called the extractions from the aloe, which had a surprisingly curative effect. Now, after many years of research, an essential contribution towards understanding the unknown active agents has been made. The results are available to patients as well as to academic medicine. Herewith the starting point has been found for a favorable influence on the course of an illness, even in such cases where the chance of recovery is slight and academic medicine is unable to put forward an acceptable concept.

The aloe healing system, for example, needs such a detailed understanding of medical indications that it is important for the afflicted person to be made familiar with the basis of the therapy.

Above all, it appears to be important to point the way which research and application have gone in order to confirm the scientific findings. The first step on the path toward discovery was the establishement of tissue therapy.

* Professor Vladimir Petrowitsch FILATOW
  Feb. 28, 1875 to Oct. 30, 1956 — Russian oculist and founder of tissue therapy

TISSUE THERAPY ACCORDING TO PROFESSOR FILATOW

AN OCULIST MAKES A DISCOVERY

Vladimir Filatow, an oculist from Odessa, received his professorship from the hands of Czar Nicholas II. Even then, he wanted more than just to practice ophthalmology within the boundaries of the scientific knowledge of his time. He felt a strong urge to investigate unknown territory; he could not accept the idea of something being incurable, he looked for new ways to create a unity between allopathy and treatment by natural remedies. It was only at a well-advanced age that he, based on the scientific progress of his home country, managed the break-through to which many people owe their eyesight; the breakthrough which introduced the tissue therapy that he founded.

Whereas in the West, treatment by natural remedies, homeopathic and anthroposophic therapies are seen as an alternative to academic medicine, to chemotherapy, and co-exist with dualistic professions, such as non-medical practitioner and homeopathic doctor in opposition to the academic physician, Filatow established the universality of the former therapies, also the totality of the possibilities of therapy. Trained in classic academic medicine and originally specializing in ophthalmology, he confirmed the sentence, »Whoever heals is right«, and demanded that physicians use a universality of possible therapies, in other words a dialectic unity of chemotherapy and biological medicine. Wherever the one does not help, the other must be tried. But the physician must be trained in all kinds of cures and gain experience. This was the demand that Filatow made on modern medicine. Again and again during his travels he encouraged the research of pharmaceutical botany.

In the Caucasian countries, in Siberia, he himself explored the active agents of plants, and stimulated the circle of his disciples to go on researching in this direction. Thus, with his »dialectic medicine«, with the unity of chemotherapy and biological therapies, Filatow for the first time opened the possibility to treat patients universally. His slogan is not to make the non-medical practitioner do battle against the academic physician in curing the patient, but to train the academic physician universally, so that he will be able to heal universally. Before one heals the sick people, the »sick universities«, which skip over phytotherapy almost completely, must be cured as well as the »sick health insurance companies«, which do not pay for natural remedies, even though a change of mind in this direction would save a lot of expenses.

Let us hear Filatow himself report how he chanced upon the dividing line between life and death, which in a few areas he was able to cross.

Filatow was on the way to found keratoplastics, i. e. corneal transplantation, and thus combat the white star. In the course of various phases of research, he reached interesting conclusions, which later on were to lead to completely new insights into the correlations within nature: »Frequently we are able to observe that after a while the transplanted cornea turns cloudy and the vision of the patient deteriorates. In such cases a transplantation can be repeated, but there is   no guarantee that the new cornea will not be likewise afflicted by the white star. When I examined a patient today, I saw the solution of the problem quite clearly. We know that sometimes tissue cultivated in artificial surroundings, isolated from its organism, stops growing. This happens regardless of nourishment and care. It suffices if one adds a new, homogeneous tisue culture to the old one; cellular growth will continue. I asked myself the question: what does the tiny piece of cornea constitute which is inserted into the opening that has been cut into the white star? Does it not resemble the tissue culture which multiplies in new, artificial surroundings? If it actually does, then a small piece of healthy cornea inserted into a transplantation which has turned cloudy would have to act just like a young tissue culture upon another one which has lost its ability to grow normally.

We remove the uppermost layer of the white star beside the cloudy cornea and in this place insert fresh transplantation material.«

This experience of the scientist had its own story. Filatow had noticed that after a corneal transplant, the white star around the implanted piece became transparent. Sometimes, the effect was so strong that all the rest of the cornea infected by the white star cleared up. This led to the assumption that the transplantation exerted a healing influence on the surrounding tissue. At great international congresses Filatow shared his findings with specialists from abroad, who in their scientific experiments had had the same experience without, however, drawing a conclusion for practical medicine from this. But this remarkable observation confirmed the theories of Filatow. The hypothesis reached through logical deduction, i. e. almost abstractly, was confirmed by observations of contemporaries and reports of scholars of our recent past. Thus began a series of experiments which astounded even clinicians themselves. In his calculations, Filatow had not erred: the implantation of a piece of cornea beside the cloudy area effected its former transparency. Here begins the decisive recognition: this clearing proceeded especially fast whenever the implanted corneal tissue came from a corpse and had been exposed to cold for a certain amount of time. For Filatow this posed the unanswered question: how does cold affect corneal tissue?

Since the time when this problem first arose its solution had become more and more difficult. The cornea exposed to cold displayed various qualities. For one thing, it eliminated the difference between dead and living tissue and thus enabled a fusion with the living organism; on the other hand, it accelerated the disappearance of the white star by its healing effects. During an operation, Filatow noted the following: the operation of a sick woman whose left eye was covered by the white star was imminent. Her right eye was not functioning, but had a healthy cornea. The doctor had decided to transplant this cornea into the left eye and to close the opening that would occur on the right eye with a chicken's cornea. The operation was successful. The cornea exposed to cold took hold and remained transparent for 40 days. In another case, clarity lasted for three months. As this shows, it was not easy to explore a state of facts which manifested itself in such various ways. The most surprising fact was this: the cold, which normally has a paralyzing effect on living tissue, proved curative here. The experience of millennia, however, proved something else. A cooling off of the human body decreases its resistance and leads to various afflictions.

Filatow had not been able to penetrate the essence of those powers that he had awakened to life. Nevertheless, he was on the way to recognizing the mysterious effect of forces which he later called biogenic stimulators.

What he had discovered in the first phase and found confirmed over and over again was surprising enough, but did not yet permit a scientific explanation. The scientist saw how in the cornea from a corpse that had been exposed to cold, the cells kept multiplying, and there was an exchange of gases. As long as these processes did not cease, the qualities of the cornea remained intact. It was difficult to believe, but true: in the corneal tissue that had been cooled to two degrees above freezing the division of cells continued. This contradicted the generally held opinion which stated that such a process at such low temperatures was impossible.

Did these peculiarities of development possibly originate only from the condition of isolated tissue? Was it not possible that the cornea, extracted from lifeless organism, had contained similar qualities before refrigeration? For a long time properties of life of isolated tissues and organs, their ability to live and to multiply, were carefully examined. The famous Russian pharmacologist Krawkow had been able to keep an amputated finger sensitive to medicaments for months. Another researcher exposed a piece of salivary gland of a rabbit to cold and was able to keep it alive for a month.

In every case the cold had a paralyzing influence on the normal functions of the isolated tissue and slowed down the division of cells decisively. For any further research, however, a hypothesis was needed, a prospective explanation of those processes which were connected with the refrigeration of the corneal tissue, and Filatow too made use of a hypothesis.

The train of thought of his hypothesis ran as follows: *Augenärzte warze*

In all probability, under the influence of the cold the cornea developed substances which had a salutary influence on the patient. As the transplanted cornea was not absorbed, but grew on, and as from this only a negligible amount of that substance was able to get into the bloodstream, the idea seemed plausible that this substance possessed extraordinary biological activity. Not every extract contained in such negligible quantities, moreover diluted in blood, would be able to retain its peculiar qualities. It appeared as if the cornea exuded a whole stream of healing substances into the white star. As a consequence, the transplantation of a tiny piece of dead cornea exerted a curative influence on the white cataracts, arrested the clouding of the cornea and made it transparent. Thus, through Filatow's work, a means was given into the hands of clinicians of reviving dead tissue to new life. Here, in fact, Filatow touched the borderline between life and death. The results did not let him rest. He was convinced that from these successes a direct path must lead to an extremely important discovery. Filatow summed up his reflections: »The white star is the consequence of a corneal disease. A piece of dead cornea which is implanted into the white star or into the cloudy cornea blots out this disease. How about making use of this curative effect of the transplantation and trying to heal other eye-diseases by this means? And would it not be possible some day to use this method for various other diseases?«

Filatow decided to test his hypothesis. He chose a patient of 16 years, Anisia Patoka. An extremely acute inflammation of the cornea caused the girl unbearable pain. Her blood-shot eyes kept running constantly. This torture had lasted for three months already. Anisia cried and wept, she begged for help, but what were the doctors to do? Congenital syphilis — the cause of her suffering — could not always be cured, let alone immediately.

The imminent operation caused great anticipation in Filatow's clinic and, as before, the conversations in the office of the scientist were animated and passionate.

»Had we not better transplant a fresh cornea this time instead of a dead one?« one physician suggested. »A fresh one?« Filatow asked in surprise. »Are you afraid the dead one might have less of an effect than a living one?«

»At the beginning I would rather make use of a proven means«, was the answer.

»For a start«, Filatow remarked ironically, »I am using a more effective means. As long as we ophthalmologists have been transplanting the corneas of living people, the clearing-up of cataract tissue around the healthy piece of cornea was relatively rare. Only dead cornea conserved by cold caused this result more frequently.«

Filatow abided by his intention to test his new idea on the operating table. He extracted a piece of inflamed cornea from his patient's eye and put a dead one in its place. On the following day the girl was able to open her eyes, and on the third day she even managed to find her way to the bandaging room unaided. The exceedingly tiny amount of the substance which had found its way from the cornea into the organism had eliminated the acute inflammation.

The consecutive operations brought the experimentator complete satisfaction. Within short periods of time corneal inflammations that had been persisting for years, were cured, and the progression of various diseases was abruptly halted.

Soon the experiments were to be extended. Herewith Filatow based his work on a textbook by Professor Baer, one of whose epigraphs runs as follows: »Whatever influences the whole, also influences a part. Whatever influences a part, also influences the whole. Whatever influences the organism, also influences the eye, and vice versa, whatever influences the eye, also influences the organism.«

Here we already have an essential starting point for modern universal medicine which Filatow made the task of his life and which he was to lead into a new dimension. The first thing that Filatow was able to ascertain was the distinctive characteristic of dead skin to influence he human organism in various ways. In one case the transplantation eliminated an inflammation, in others it restored the elasticity of the sclera, stimulated the function of the connective tissue, healed bad scars and made the cornea transparent again. Filatow doubted that these qualities should be inherent in dead corneal tissue only. Which reasons could there be for nature to preserve a special privilege for this tissue? The substances that formed in the refrigerated tissue from corpses must likewise develop in other tissue. Was it conceivable that everything living in an organism developed new qualities through the cold? If this was true, then it must be the way to solve the mystery of those substances which also accumulated in dead tissue. Further experience showed that ailing organs did not necessarily have to be cured with related tissue. The effect was the same if some liquid extract from any tissue which had been exposed to cold was injected into the patients. Blood, spinal liquid as well as the contents of the eye, exposed to cold, displayed healing effects when injected under the skin.

Filatow turned to plants. For a long time the aloe, the Biblical plant, repeatedly and mysteriously mentioned in the Old Testament, had interested him; he also knew its effects from popular medicine in Asia. He ventured a first experiment. Filatow separated aloe leaves from the plant and for about ten days kept them without light at a temperature of 3 degrees above zero (3° C); afterwards the leaves were crushed, and the juice thus extracted was injected under the skin of a patient — after this had been tried out on animals. The extract had the same effect on the disease as dead tissue inserted into the cell structure.

Now Filatow could have said full of conviction:

Any deterioration of the conditions of life, whether of animal or plant organism, if the degree of deprivation does not pass a certain limit, causes a kind of emergency in this organism which sets in motion complicatet changes:

new life regulators emerge.

Last doubts dissolved when Flatow boiled the leaves of agaves into juice, filled it into test tubes and put it into the autoklav (steam pot) at a temperature of 120 degrees Celsius for one hour. After this process there was no trace of protein left in the juice, but when injected into the organism of the patient it worked like freshly extracted juice from a preserved leaf. Preserved dead tissue as well as green leaves which for a while were kept without light and afterwards in the autoklav exposed to a temperature of about 120 degrees Celsius not only retained their qualities, but even intensified them.

Soon afterwards much of the nature of the stimulators came to light: it was shown that they were neither proteins nor enzymes. The ones as well as the others are destroyed by such high temperatures. When a tiny piece of tissue preserved in the autoklav was inserted into a culture of isolated tissue in which the division of cells had already slowed down, intensive growth resumed.

The stimulators did not disappear from a waterey extract of aloe even when the extract was boiled, evaporated and reliquified.

Now this liquid contained neither protein nor hormones nor even salts, but the stimulators were there, and the healing properties of the extract were intact. From experiment to experiment, from successful cure to successful cure it became clearer to Filatow that it was not the cornea itself nor the extract in the material sense which effected the healing process, but the biogenic stimulators contained therein. What are biogenic stimulators and how do they work?

Filatow proceeded empirically according to the slogan »He who heals in right.« It interested him only as a physician. With his magnificent cures he had raised medicine onto a new, heretofore unattained level. As a scientist he contented himself with stating that the biogenic stimulators were based on active agents of an unknown nature.

But in order to apply the broad indications of Filatow's tissue therapy, which revolutionizes no less than the whole practical medicine as well as the therapies of hospitals and clinics, in Western medicine, the scientific criteria valid here make it necessary to define the character of biogenic stimulators and prove their working mechanisms.

This has now been done.

The Arbeitsgemeinschaft Grundlagenforschung für biologische Medizin (The Study Group of Basic Research for Biological Medicine) has proved the biogenic stimulators and developed from this a biological complex-therapy, which can now be used without restraint.

ON THE NATURE OF BIOGENIC STIMULATORS

Let us remember how Professor Filatow explains his tissue therapy: »I have developed a tissue therapy in the sense of a non-specific stimulation therapy. It makes use of certain active agents of an unexplained nature, which develop in plant and animal tissues when preserved in cold or darkness. These biogenic stimulators also develop in the tissues of the agave and the aloe.«

In plant organisms als well as in tissues surviving separate from them, under the influence of harmful, but non-lethal external factors, a biochemical restructuring takes place, whose consequence is the formation of compounds of high biological activity.

The aloe compounds belong to the group of non-specific stimulants of the physiological functions of the organism. Strengthening the powers of adaptation and resistance of a patient through the aloe therapy makes it possible to use specific drugs to greater effect.

The complicated biochemical structure causes the unusually broad pharmacological spectrum and the wide influence on the function of practically all organs and systems of the human body.

The latest research has shown that the aloe compounds, as far as they are biostimulated, are somehow related to the organism in the same way as all tissue compounds of Filatow's method are. Therefore they have a low toxic content and are almost free of side effects.

THE WORKING MECHANISM OF BIOGENIC STIMULATORS

Biogenic stimulators from the aloe function via the central nervous system. Experiments concerning the influence of aloe compounds on the central nervous system have the following purposes:

1. Establishing the role of the central nervous system within the working mechanism of the aloe compounds.
2. Practical advice concerning the application of aloe compounds in clinical practice.

Already in the first experiments the influence of the aloe extract on the central nervous system was proven. In his analysis of various aspects of the activity of aloe compounds, the Russian physician S. M. Pawlenko als early as 1953 ascribes great importance to the reflexive influences via the central nervous system.

When judging the effect of aloe compounds on the functional state of the central nervous system, many scientists used the method of conditional reflexes.

Most researchers noted that the aloe therapy causes a delay of the latent period of reflexive reactions, an increase of the duration of reflexes, a decrease of the intensity of conditional reflexes to the point of their complete disappearance. This allows us to call it an intensification of the preventive processes in the central nervous system.

The important part played by the central nervous system within the working mechanism of the aloe compounds is confirmed by the observations of the pharmaco-dynamic changes of the aloe compounds when the functional state of the central nervous system changes.

Experiments with rabbits proved that drug-induced sleep of different intesity changes the influence of aloe compounds on many biochemical processes and on the functions of the connective tissue considerably.

For the understanding of the working mechanism of aloe extracts the examination of the activity of the enzyme system in the brain is of special importance. Under the influence of aloe extract an increase of activity of some oxydation enzymes in the cerebrum of test animals was noted: zytochromoxydasis, dehydrasis, succinathydrogenasis, glycerophosphatdehydrogenasis, glutamat-dehydrogenasis, and succino-oxydasis.

In medium therapeutic doses aloe extract increased the activity of cholinesterasis in the cerebral cortex of test animals, in their sub-cortex, thalamus, hypo-thalamus and in the extended marrow of white rats. The application of larger doses of biogenic stimulants however decreased the activity of the cholinesterasis in all examined parts of the brain. Furthermore, the experiments showed in general that the activity in the examined structures and organs changes considerably on the third, ninth, sixteenth, and twentyfirst days after the first application. The main tendency herein was the increase of activity of the above-mentioned enzymes. Based of the results of the experiments, Russian physicians were soon able to give practical advice concerning the use of the aloe extract. In the aloe therapy, the general condition of the patient's nervous system, as well as his disposition have to be closely monitored. The aloe therapy is also effective with such afflictions in whose pathogenesis an irritation of the higher parts of the central nervous system with the formation of a persistent irritation center can be assumed, such as ulcus diseases, angiospasms, contractions, hypertension. The retardation of the cerebral cortex during the aloe therapy is judged by the leading researchers to be a therapeutic protective retardation; this underlines the usefulness of aloe compounds in practical medicine.

In the face of the positive effect of the aloe extract on the functioning of the central nervous system of aging people, i.e. the sedative, calming effect, the use of aloe extract in geriatrics is to be recommended. It is here that Russian physicians can claim constant success. The proven intensification of Hexenal-sleep through aloe compounds with old test animals makes it possible to decrease the doses of barbiturates in geriatric practice. This is of special practical importance, because older people often take barbiturates for sleeping problems which may be caused by intoxication phenomena.

For the restoration of failing locomotive functions and for the stimulation of the regenerative processes within the central nervous system aloe compounds can be especially recommended. The experiments conducted with spinal marrow in clinical tests showed an increase of the regenerative processes, for instance the restoration of impulse conduction across the bisected part of marrow.

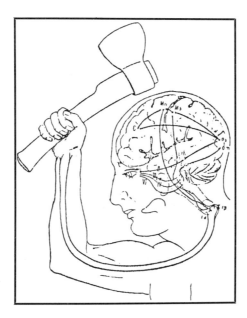

Bechterew's schematic representation of impulse conduction during a phase of work

The aloe therapy has an indisputable effect in the treatment of neuralgia, causalgia and phantom pains. The Russian physicians Woljanski and Kurako, both disciples of Filatow, used aloe extract in the treatment of lumbal-sacral radiculitides of discogenic, traumatic, infectious and catarrhal aetiology from 1972 on and concluded that the therapy in connection with analgetics guarantees a rapid lessening of the pain syndrome and recovery in case of motoric disturbances (especially with paralytic sciatica).

Filatow himself stressed that the lessening and eventual elimination of pain in peripheral nervous diseases is a general characteristic of the working mechanism of the aloe therapy. This manifests itself in a resorption of the inflammation-infiltrates and in a softening of scar tissue around the afflicted nerves.

The aloe therapy is effective in the treatment of inflamed spinal marrow and its skins. It effects an improvement of the condition of a patient with spinal arachnoiditis, i.e. the dangerous meningitis, as well as the cure of myelitis. The aloe extract therapy has an especially salutary influence on the functioning of the aging organism. Thus a decrease of asthenia symptoms and a considerable increase of spiritual capacity with elderly and even very old patients could be noted.

Clinical observations of 590 children with birth traumas over a long period of time have shown the following results: The children were given aloe extract in combination with vitamin B 12. In all cases an extraordinarily beneficial effect on the growing process of the brain was observed.

In experiments with new-born animals, the above-mentioned compounds displayed a stimulating effect on the growth of the cerebral capillary as well as the resistance of cerebrovascular vessels.

All clinical data demonstrate a high biological activity of aloe extract and a decisive influence of the biogenic stimulators on the central nervous system.

Meanwhile clinical data have been made available which show that aloe extract used in the treatment of arteriosclerosis effects a noticeable lowering of the increased cholesterol level in the blood and keeps the lecithin-cholesterol coefficient on a higher level. These facts were confirmed in a case of arteriosclerosis of vessels of the extremities. Under the influence of this therapy a decrease and, in many cases, a disappearance of pains in the extremities, as well as improved blood circulation and a rise in skin temperature were brought about. All this led to long-lasting remissions or clinical healing with recovery of the ability to work. Aloe extract is used with great success for treating inflammations and regeneration processes, especially in cases of retarded regeneration and with anemias.

Aloe has a pronounced prophylactic and therapeutic influence in cases of injuries caused by radiation damages and in cases of intoxication. The eminent German physician, Prof. Dr. Brandt, states in a treatise on tissue therapy:

»Filatow points out that the biogenic stimulators influence the whole organism; this would explain their manifold effect.«

The influence of the aloe therapy on the function of the kidney and the suprarenal gland is of great importance. With this improvement, a normalization of the processes of metabolism and the disappearance of a number of indications go hand in hand, which are caused by the intoxication of the organism by the products of an imperfect metabolism. The improved condition of the patient treated according to the aloe therapy and his own subjective impression of the effect of the therapy is, among all the changes, the most pronounced phenomenon registered in the experiments. Whereas with about half the examined patients after a series of ten injections positive changes in the vasotonia and the heart action were established by instrumental methods, the overwhelming majority of patients felt an improvement of their condition of varying degrees after one to four cures with aloe extract. Without exception these cures were administered to aging people. The changes in the condition of these people can be traced back to a considerable lessening or the disappearance of many afflictions which are characteristic of the decrepitude of the organism. Annoying pains in the joints of the extremities, in the spinal column, disappeared, sleep became normal, dizziness vanished, shortness of breath occurred more rarely. Pounding of the heart, irregular heartbeat, dullness in the legs decreased, the unpleasant taste in the mouth disappeared, and intestinal function was activated. As a result, motoric and spiritual activity, the ability to work and, with some patients, also sexual potency were restored; as a result, the general interest in life widened and intensified.

The subjective and objective changes described here, which occurred in the organism of old people under the influence of the aloe therapy, were different in intensity, duration and constancy, and to a large degree depended on the initial state of health of the patient. We have already stated that the positive effect occurs more often when in the original condition the negative functional changes of the blood circulation under physical aspects (haemodynamics) were more pronounced. The most frequent improvements occurred after the first and second injection cures. Third and fourth cures tended to be less effective. In the periods between the cures the condition usually deteriorated somewhat, but rarely down to the original level. Those researchers who used the aloe extract in geriatrics stress the necessity of an individual dosage of injections and of pauses between the cures. They come to the conclusion that the dose for older people must be smaller than for younger ones. The mechanism of the beneficent effect of the therapy on the heart circulation system is connected with an improvement of the metabolic processes in the tissues of the heart and blood vessels. A number of experimental observations proves the activation of enzymes of the heart tissue under the influence of the therapy. In these experiments an increased tissue respiration was noted. This could be judged after an increase in the activity of various enzymes.

The level of energy of cholinesterasis was substantinally increased. Under the influence of the therapy, the functional optimum of several enzymes is increased and altered. Aloe extract heightens the reflexive sensitivity and the susceptibility of the organism to a number of drugs, especially to the effect of adrenalin. A number of experimental observations prove the stimulating influence of the therapy on the function of several endocrine glands: pancreas, thyroid gland, suprarenal cortex. The therapy improves the coefficients of haemodynamics, normalizes the vasotonia; a sizable number of patients noted a decrease or disappearance of vasomotoric disturbances; angiospasms and ischaemia indications disappeared, the blood supply in tissues was increased. These changes also had a positive influence on the general condition of the wilting organism, on the character and intensity of the aging process. Therefore the aloe therapy can be recommended as an effective therapeutic and prophylactic means in geriatric medicine.

THE ALOE THERAPY AS A NEW BIOLOGICAL HEALING SYSTEM

The treatment with bio-stimulating active agents from the aloe first recommended by the Russian scientist Prof. Vladimir Filatow is a non-specific stimulation therapy. To a certain extent it resembles the working mechanisms of homeopathy. Filatow sees the aloe therapy as part of the tissue therapy that he founded in 1933. According to his school of thought, all tissue compounds are stimulants of the physiological functions of the organism; they are more effective and act physiologically in a natural way, more so than other compounds used for this purpose. The preparation of the tissues is based on the hypothesis of Filatow which says that within different organisms as well as in surviving tissues separated from them there takes place a biological transformation under the influence of harmful, but non-lethal factors, which results in the formation of biologically active compounds. Summarily this is the logic of Filatow's hypothesis. Reality proved the researcher right. Dr. Arjajew, a disciple of the famous physician, reports that numerous animal experiments and, eventually, clinical observations proved that the bio-stimulated tissues showed a more pronounced effect than the freshly procured ones. By now, tissue therapy has been applied successfully in the U.S.S.R. for many years. This method has held up in long-lasting clinical examinations. Based on this practical experience in various medical fields the indications could be concreted into tissue therapy. Nevertheless it is surprising that this biological healing system has found no, or only insufficient, attention within so-called Western medicine. The reason is simple, but not persuasive. In Russia, the principle »He who heals is right« has always been valid. Therefore the main object was to heal with a new therapy, whereas it seemed less urgent to procure the scientific proof for its effectiveness and the exact process of the working mechanisms. Since, however, the academic medicine of the West prescribes that a new therapy can be applied only after the criteria of the working mechanisms have been successfully proven − which happens to be the basic problem of homeopathy! − it was now a matter of prime importance to clear up the nature of the biogenic stimulators in the sense of a scientific proof; only this way was it possible to put the new biological healing system to practical use.

Whereas Prof. Filatow did not lift the cloak of mystery from the biogenic stimulators, the first Western exploratory attempts turned out to be failures. This precluded the possibilities of healing millions of patients by means of the new therapy systems. In this context it is of great importance to state in the interest of the necessary breakthrough of tissue therapy, especially the aloe healing system, in which ways and with which results Western academic medicine has confronted the new therapy system.

Among the first professionals who took tissue therapy and the hypothesis concerning the biogenic stimulators seriously at an early time was Dr. Max Brandt, a physician and academic teacher renowned far beyond German borders, who taught at the Free University of Berlin. From the Institute for Eastern Europe of the above-mentioned university he edited a series of medical publications in which he also thoroughly reported on tissue therapy and raised the question of biogenic stimulators.

These reports demonstrate how in long years the medical school after Prof. Filatow progressed from the success of tissue therapy toward the less complicated aloe therapy through practical experience. It is these representations which will not only convince the expert reader, but also the patient, of the scientific credibility of the indicational claims as well as the reported successes.

The starting point in the tissue therapy is to be found in the cornea transplantations by Filatow. Whereas in the eye-clinic of Odessa about 1000 successful cornea transplants were carried out prior to 1949, according to the report of Dr. Brandt, 4064 transplantations of this kind were performed in the U.S.S.R. by July, 1951; the result was fantastic: 65 % of the patients regained their vision. In only 43 cases did the coneal transplant turn cloudy. In this connection it was discovered that through the transplantation of small pieces of tissue, retarded growth was again stimulated. This stimulation of growth is ascribed to the effect of certain substances which are called desmones. The latter method, however, was not successful in the long run. The initial assessments were correct, and Filatow ventured on new paths: he started transplanting dead cornea which had been preserved at a temperature of 2 − 4 degrees C. for two or three days. The result was promising. Not only did the transplanted piece of dead cornea remain clear, but also the original, cloudy cornea around it began to clear up. Dr. Brandt comments, »During the refrigeration there presumably occurred an accumulation of unknown active agents. Those however do not seem to be of a specific nature, because histologically non-identical tissue has the same effect . . . «. In his therapeutic experiments, Filatow then started using plant tissues, after he had gained corresponding knowledge from working with agaves (agava americana). From here finally the theory of the biogenic stimulators was developed. Dr. Max Brandt describes them as follows, »The tissue parts separated from the host organ and placed under unfavorable conditions are biochemically transformed and develop substances which increase the vital reactions and promote healing. In these cases, it is not necessary to perform an implantation, as injections can produce the same effect.«

Later it was noted that the biogenic healing agents of aloe arborescens are even stronger than those of the agave. With this knowledge, however, the biogenic stimulators were still not established, and thus the scientific proof was lacking. Nevertheless it is of interest that Dr. Brandt was the first to start chemical examination of the biogenic stimulators. His research proved the following substances: »Oxalic and succinic acids, malic and tartaric acids, unsaturated, aromatic fatty and phenol acids.«

This enumeration of substances, however, is not a sufficient description of the nature of the biogenic stimulators. The listed substances, at least the essential ones, are part of the citric acid cycle of the human organism. The citric acid cycle is responsible for the consumption of carbohydrates, proteins etc. as the basis of energy balance.

The conclusion from the aptly described examinations of substances leads up to principal contradictions. The established substances belonging to the citric acid cycle of the human organism do not affect the central nervous system, because for this, minute chemical, high-molecular substances are required. But those substances form, like the acids named by Dr. Brandt, under the same conditions as the tissue parts separated from the host organ and placed under unfavorable conditions, where they undergo a biochemical transformation.

For a while the author of this publication presumed in the course of his research that the biogenic stimulators were hormone-like, high-molecular substances, as hormones and similar systems are unprovable with the present means of measuring, because they are destroyed, whereas on the other hand they have the same effect; in other words, the biogenic stimulators are more than the substances named by Dr. Brandt.

Above all, this is proven by their practical application:

Aloe is available in the pharmacy in different forms of administration, i.e. pills, homeopathic injections and dilutions. They are administered as laxatives, as a means of intestinal regulation. If from the outset the aloe contained those substances from the active agents of the biogenic stimulators, without any interference in the tissue organization of the plants through the cutting off of leaves, the conventionally available aloe medicine would have to satisfy the same demands of indication as stated in this publication. As we know, this is not the case, as these aloe compounds act as a purgative only.

Summarizing, we have to say that the biogenic stimulators, first applied by the school of Filatow, whose nature has now been explained, come into being exclusively through biochemical reorganization, i.e. when the »tissue parts separated from the host organ and placed under unfavorable conditions develop those substances«, which influence the vital reactions of the organism.

These substances are high-molecular, therefore the extreme dilution, they are desmones, similar to desmo-enzymes, firmly established in the cell, but they survive the measuring conditions; their isolation produces so-called heteroglycanes.

They have the effect of a co-enzyme system and can be seen as »co-desmone principle«.

THE INDIVIDUAL DISEASES AND THEIR CURES

ADDISON'S DISEASE

This disease, formerly considered rare, but nowadays occurring more frequently, is an insufficiency of the suprarenal cortex.

As with all diseases that have to do with man's immune system, this affliction has hardly been researched. Its name is derived from the English physician Thomas Addison (1793 – 1860).

It is specifically the increase of the number of cases which indicates that the development toward high civilization with its inherent stress on the immune system at different levels, especially the psyche, fosters such diseases. The consequence, not the cause, of Addison's Disease is the hormone production emanating from the suprarenal gland effecting the destruction of at least nine tenths of the gland.

As of today, academic medicine has not explored the connection between the suprarenal gland and the other so-called endocrine glands. The author is of the opinion that there is a close connection with the thyroid gland, likewise an endocrine gland. In the case of thyrotoxicosis, metabolic disturbances follow. With Addison's Disease, the cause is to be found in metabolic disturbances in the electrolytic and carbohydrate metabolism.

There is an excessive fallout of adrenalin. This is an essential characteristic of a disease of the suprarenal gland. Other reasons can be inflammatory processes and degenerative changes (vessel stoppages, lues). These comments are meant to stimulate the exploration of the interdependence with thyroid function.

We know the following symptoms:

Excessive fatigue after a short time, limpness to the point of exhaustion, weight loss, inflammation of oral membranes, muscle weakness, anaemia, backache, listlessness, the whole tonicity is disturbed.

This disease is a consequence of considerable disturbances within the immune system, so that the therapy must concentrate on strengthening the immune system.

The aloe-injection therapy for the first time presents a natural possibility of healing and strengthening the immune system. Instructions are as follows:

On 30 consecutive days one injection each of 1 ml is to be administered subcutaneously into the thigh, preferably in the early morning hours, followed by 15 minutes of rest. After this series leave an interval of 30 days, then follows the second phase of therapy with another 30 injections in a daily sequence.

After one year the cure should be repeated.

THE FEAR OF AIDS

At a satanic speed a disease is spreading, which poses unsolved problems to science; its name, AIDS, is the abbreviation of »Acquired Immune Deficiency Syndrome«. This is a rather general and temporary description, which shows the complete impotence of academic medicine in the face of this virus disease. The name AIDS was coined by the renowned discoverer of the so-called HTLV III virus, Professor Dr. Robert Gallo (U.S.A.). It is a striking fact that up to now homosexuals with a high rate of promiscuity constitute the majority of patients (about 75 %); the rest are drug addicts, hemophiliacs as well as people infected by blood transfusion.

It seems to have originated in Central Africa; Haiti is strongly affected, and the spread from the U.S.A. across Europe and Asia proceeds at a frightening speed, so that it has to be called an epidemic.

Renowned virologists throughout the world are investigating AIDS intensively. They are trying to discover a serum, but as yet the prospects are poor. As the British virologist Dr. Angus Dalgleish (Chester Beaty Laboratories, London) describes the situation:

»A serum must alarm the immune system of the body to search for a particular virus, in much the same way as the police search for a stolen car with the help of its license number.«

But now the above-mentioned scientist has discovered that the AIDS virus is able to keep changing its chemical make-up, so that finding and identifying it is impossible. Consequently, various syndromes appear, which develop or are favored by the disturbance of the immune system through the AIDS virus; this is especially true of infectious diseases, among them an infectious variety of pneumonia. For an AIDS patient an otherwise relatively harmless disease such as angina, can be fatal.

The serum which has not yet been found is probably not the complete solution to the problem. Above all, the object must be to strengthen the immune system disturbed by the AIDS virus. The author of this publication goes even further: only after the weakening of the immune system does the virus have a chance to trigger the disease. It has been noted that the disease does not break out with every homosexual who carries the virus. A disease does not break out as long as the immune system functions reasonably well. The patients have not been well enough differentiated as to whether the homosexuals had steady partners or were promiscuous. Such an analysis would demonstrate that especially with promiscuous patients the disease becomes serious. We get closer to the root of things if we investigate the concrete situation of those people, because it differs considerably from those homosexuals with steady partners. The promiscuous person lives in constant fear of discovery with his ever-changing, short-lived intimate contacts; during the fulfillment of his wishful fantasies he finds himself for a few moments at a very high level of excitement, a kind of super stress, without harmonious development of the intimate relationship and without a fulfilling ebbing of a close partnership. In this phase of anxiety − excitement − super stress, an excessive amount of adrenalin is produced, that important hormone originating in the suprarenal gland. The repeated stress through anxiety weakens the immune system to the point where the AIDS virus in blood infected by violent contacts can penetrate unopposed, so that any infection may fatally weaken the patient.

If the group of AIDS patients is analyzed objectively, the question arises why the inhabitants of Haiti of both sexes, even children, why part of the population of the Central African Republic are especially prone to be afflicted by the AIDS virus − if this is supposed to be an exclusive disease of homosexuals. These groups with different life styles must have similar original dispositions − independent of their sexual preferences − which create the conditions for the AIDS virus. In connection with poor hygienic conditions it is the anxiety that the especially afflicted groups of people have in common: anxiety of all types. With the promiscuous homosexuals it is the stress of their particular situation and the panic of discovery; with the Haitians and Central Africans − both from the poorhouses of the world, which is symptomatic − it is the continuous struggle for existence, consequences of poverty, also of whole generations with corresponding genetic material, the daily fear of tomorrow!

Anxiety does not lead to infection, but under the conditions of radically restricted immune powers it leads to the breakdown of the body's defenses.

The fact that an AIDS patient has to be told that he is afflicted with a disease or an epidemic whose cause is unknown and which has no prospects of being cured, leads to another mentally conditioned restriction of the body's defenses and the will to resist. The prospect of being able to undergo a cure to rebuild the immune system, however slowly, leads to encouragement, to mobilizing the last powers of resistance.

This is an essential platform for the therapy. These psychological findings should not be forgotten during the work with AIDS patients in their difficult situation.

In this context, prophylactic medicine is of eminent importance. A realist will admit that certain life styles conditioned by inheritance and instinctive desires can hardly be changed. We must help these people by educational work concerning special dangers of infection through certain practices, which should include prophylactic measures. This is the more important, as AIDS can have an incubation time of several years. At any rate, timely application of aloe extract can favorably influence the disease in its early stages.

Favorable expectations concerning a therapy with aloe injections are based on the fact that almost 50 % of the patients that had been treated with aloe developed irregular antibodies in their blood.

Irregular antibodies, however, are immune antibodies. These are of eminent importance in the battle against the AIDS virus.

The following therapy is recommended to the physicians concerned:

> At first aloe extract is injected into the thigh, subcutaneously, once a day for 30 consecutive days, 1 ml per injection. After 30 days there follows an interval without injections. Afterwards, another cure phase of 30 days with one daily injection of 1 ml each. This injection cure is to be repeated once a year for the following three years according to the above-mentioned instructions.

We are at the very beginning of AIDS research. Whichever results science may reach in the future, the immune condition must be the basis of all considerations. It is to be noted that a weakened immune system will be further weakened by the AIDS virus, at worst with fatal results. Every therapy must begin with the rebuilding of the immune powers. A platitude? If one analyzes the treatment of AIDS patients up to now it has to be noted that the immune condition **before** the AIDS infection, and its background have hardly been taken into account.

The parallels to cancer should become apparent!

AIDS — THE LATEST STAGE OF RESEARCH

Under heading »5« of the information sheet published by the German Ministry of Health, the following basic advice is given in the chapter »What You Should Do in Case of an Infection«: **»Strengthen your defenses!«**

This recommendation can only be welcomed. It concerns the immune system. Also the priority is correctly stated. Strengthening the immune powers has absolute preference over the development of a vaccine. This is required by the working mechanism of the AIDS viruses. American scientists are convinced that the AIDS viruses constantly change their »uniform« (this is a simplified explanation), so that the active agents of a vaccination do not, or only partially, expose them. Prof. Dr. Robert Schooley from Boston noted in 1985 that the AIDS viruses invade the central nervous system and use it as a kind of refuge. As a consequence, various diseases of the central nervous system, such as an especially dangerous form of meningitis, are triggered. The American scientist noted that the blood-brain barrier is broken by the AIDS virus. Normally it is this blood-brain barrier which protects the nerve cells against the invasion of noxious substances, viruses and bacteria. This poses an additional danger to the infected person. Prof. Schooley, »The AIDS virus is able to multiply within the cells of the central nervous system. Therefore any treatment of the lethal viruses must penetrate the blood-brain barrier. Most medicaments are not able to do this.«

In connection with these statements and prognoses it is of special importance to accomplish the task with an active agent developed in a natural way to protect the central nervous system and keep it intact. This task is best accomplished by the aloe healing system with its injection cures. Plainly speaking, if in the future a vaccine should be discovered which actually combats the virus, its effect will be greater if the immune system has been strengthened before by an aloe treatment, whose mechanism works via the central nervous system.

The American Cancer Institute reports that it will probably be impossible to develop a general vaccine against the AIDS virus, because it does not have a uniform genetic structure and thus varies from person to person.

The latest findings of research confirm the attack of the AIDS viruses directed against the brain and spinal marrow. Researchers of Massachusetts General Hospital in Boston have proved the presence of the virus in the brain and spinal marrow of AIDS patients suffering from neurological disturbances.

The »New England Journal of Medicine« adds that it is almost impossible to get medicaments in adequate concentrations beyond the blood-brain barrier to the spot which is essential for combating the AIDS virus. These statements are no mere hypotheses. Meanwhile one scientist has succeeded in proving the existence of the AIDS virus in the brain. At the international AIDS congress in Naples, Prof. Joseph Melnick from Houston, Texas, showed pictures made by an electron microscope of brain cells which were infected by the AIDS virus and had multiplied there. In its issue of December 16, 1985, the German medical journal »Der Apotheker« adds:

»The pictures by the electron microscope depict tissue samples extracted from AIDS patients . . . With the help of the electron microscope various tissue samples (kidney, lymphonodes, bone marrow, brain) of altogether 80 AIDS patients have been examined for more than two and a half years. Among other things it was found that the AIDS virus infects not only the white, but also the gray cells in the brain. Moreover, AIDS viruses were found in the blood cells of the cerebrospinal fluid, which also courses through the brain.«

All these terrifying statements call upon us to make immune therapy the therapy of the future. Above all, research should not pass by the potential of active agents which nature itself offers. The possibilities opened up by the active agents from the aloe point the way. With new diseases one gets the impression that at the beginning the research is conducted within the means of chemotherapy only, whereas medicinal botany is completely neglected. Dr. Veronica Carstens, a competent and courageous physician, says in an interview of June 16, 1985, for the newspaper »Welt am Sonntag« – this is an interesting and important impulse: »A few years ago an American biologist went to Peru. She lived among Indians. There she made a remarkable discovery. The means for family planning seemed to grow on bushes. When the women ate the leaves of a certain bush, they did not become pregnant. In the jungle, according to the U.S. biologist, there also grows a contraceptive – the leaves of another bush. To be sure, this is a fascinating story. Up to now, no pharmaceutical firm has found it worthwhile to pursue this.«

These impulses should stimulate research and medical science to explore the idea of medicinal botany. The results that this can produce are shown by the aloe healing system, which for the first time has been dealt with at great length in this publication, and also by the well-known plant echinacea. Popular medicine has always maintained that this plant contains an active agent which stregthens the defenses of the organism. In fact, under certain conditions biogenic stimulators can be developed from echinacea which resemble the aloe and have a similar effect. In the above-mentioned interview, Dr. Carstens adds: »Now it has been proved at the University of Munich that the number of white corpuscles, which promote immunity, rises under the influence of echinacea. At a low dosage it is especially effective. This is impressive. Every physician should be open toward such developments.« This should also be true for the AIDS research, which must not exhaust itself in the search for a new vaccine, but be open toward all conceivable possibilities for the strengthening of the immune system.

Lately the discussions among professionals concerning the causes for the emergence of the AIDS virus have become more and more controversial. This publication intends to add only a brief statement by shedding light on those conditions of life which cause diseases, but are often underestimated. It is not genetic engineering by scientists which triggered the AIDS virus, but, in the last consequence, it is social conditions. In the Central African Republic as well as among the tribes of other African countries there is a species of monkeys called green monkeys (cercopeticus aetiops). These monkeys congregate wherever they find refuse. Garbage dumps are their favorite haunts. In their search for things to eat they compete with people of the poorest sort. In this battle for survival between man and beast there have been contacts with the green monkey, which among other populations have been the original hosts of the AIDS virus, but manage well on account of their immune apparatus. These contacts are easily conceivable, e.g. in the form of monkey bites, or monkey meat eaten. In the new carrier, man, the AIDS virus found an especially weakened immune system caused by need and deprivation, by deficiency diseases and profound anxiety. We know that an infection triggers the disease only if the body's defenses cannot cope with the virus.

The frequently blurred facts concerning the origin of the AIDS virus should point out the close connection between disease and social conditions.

The latest research of AIDS, above all the one concerning the penetration of the virus into the central nervous system, confirms the value of the aloe healing system as one of the major therapy alternatives. The bio-stimulated aloe-extract injections are a relief army!

ALOE AND CHEMOTHERAPY

The therapy based on the aloe healing system creates a favorable basis for bridging the dualism between treatment by natural remedies and academic chemotherapy. In fact, the tissue therapy with aloe is an ideal bridge between various healing methods. We cannot emphasize strongly enough that an important precondition for this has to be provided by academic medicine itself. It must open up at long last toward the findings concerning the healing properties and protective substances of plants. A considerable, and growing, number of compounds prescribed in doctors' offices contain plant substances either exclusively or partially, but the docter has not had adequate contact with medicinal botany in his medical studies. Thus he does not know the indications of his prescriptions – at least not from his studies at the university – so that the connection between the specific organism of the plants with the human organism often remains unknown to him. Phytotherapy, i.e. healing through plants, medicinal botany, as well as biochemistry according to Dr. Schüssler should have their place on an equal footing with chemical therapies in the curriculum of the universities. If we do not close our eyes to the truth we must find the situation of treatment by natural remedies within our society simply grotesque. They are used by non-medical practitioners and a minority of natural-cure doctors, both looked down upon as outsiders that are at best tolerated. But the facts are not taught at universities! »The grotesque situation of natural remedies is characterized by the grotesque situation of academic medicine«, because the latter objects to healing practices as scientifically unproven or even as unscientific – for the sole reason that its own criteria of examination do not suffice, being incomplete, to confront scientifically, say, a medical category based on experience such as homeopathy. The one-sided reliance of our academic medicine on quantitative scientific criteria is the main obstacle. What is missing is dialectics. Thus is has become frozen in its tracks. In practical consequence, academic medicine as an established science simply attacks the other, as yet non-established, sciences with all means available, even though it lacks the instruments for a scientific controversy. It is a striking fact that the attacks against medical categories based on experience are usually not led by practicing doctors who have contact with patients, but by forensic doctors, pathologists, doctors at medical institutes, and professors.

The inherent contradiction of our academic medicine in theory and in practice clearly points up the task of pharmacies. Every pharmacy, visible for every patient, displays its universal field of activity: allopathy, homeopathy, biochemistry. So here they are assembled, the compounds of chemotherapy as well as the ones of natural healing methods. To be sure, the latter ones have their place on the shelves of an academically educated pharmacist, but at the universities there is no room for teaching the scientific findings and proven information concerning those compounds available under pharmaceutical law. According to the logic of conservative universities, the pharmacist keeps medicine available which, at least by the limited standard of knowledge at many universities, cannot be listed as medicine. As Wilhelm Busch used to say, »that whatever must not be cannot be . . . «

Present-day knowledge concerning the working mechanism of the aloe, however, shows that the human organism proves a connection between chemotherapy and natural-cure methods. In Russia, aloe in a special form of application was first used as universal medicine: the watery extract from the stimulated juice of aloe leaves produced in a special procedure is injected as medicine for various indications. In the U.S.S.R. itself this medicament is sold as »extractum aloes«, extract of the plant. No further definition is given. In other words, this extract is prescribed by doctors, it is used in hospitals and clinics. An analysis of the extract, however, shows that it is a homeopathic compound, because the plant extract is diluted to the homeopathic potency of D 2.

This proves that one individual extract can at the same time be an allopathic as well as a homeopathic compound. This fact shows how meaningless the confrontation between allopathy and homeopathy is, and it makes clear that the attacks by academic medicine on homeopathy are meaningless for the patients. To them it is not important by which method they are treated, but to be cured.

The aloe therapy, however, does not only point the way on a purely academic level toward an integration of allopathy and homeopathic categories, but proves to be a veritable bridge to chemotherapy.

It has been clinically proven that within the patients the aloe therapy can considerably increase the powers of adaptation and defense. This makes it possible to apply all specifically directed medical means, including chemotherapy, to maximum effect. The dosage of chemical as well as natural compounds with most afflictions is lower if the therapy with the scientifically directed medicaments is preceded by an aloe treatment. In this context we must remind the reader of the working mechanism of the aloe compounds – they are stimulators of the physiological functions of the organism; their complicated structure explains the unusually broad pharmacological spectrum and the manifold effect on the functions of all organs and systems of the organism.

Therefore the aloe therapy should not be reserved for non-medical practitioners, but must be a stimulation for academic medicine and practicing doctors alike to combine chemotherapy with the biological healing systems described in this publication. This would really be a turning point for the benefit of the patients!

The social effect would be a considerable saving of expenses, because fewer chemical compounds can be used to greater effect; and on an individual basis it would mean a reduction of chemical applications to the necessary minimum.

ANAEMIA

Anaemia, a typical deficiency disease with lack of iron in the organism, keeps spreading. The number of children afflicted is striking.

The paleness so characteristic of this deficiency is the consequence of a decrease of blood pigment. The importance of red blood corpuscles is demonstrated by their task: they transport the oxygen. The waste matter produced by the metabolism is transported by the blood liquid, as are the defensive substances and nutritional substances of the organism. The red color of the blood corpuscles is produced by haemoglobin. This coloring contains the iron so indispensable for us; thus haemoglobin guarantees the constant supply of oxygen.

In case of a deficient oxygen supply with anaemia it is especially the heart muscle that suffers, so that cramps, constrictions, even shortness of breath occur. As the brain does not receive a sufficient blood supply, head-ache, typical of anaemia, early exhaustion, buzzing in the ears, numbness in the limbs, and insomnia set it.

A frequent variety of anaemia is greensickness, also called chlorosis. It occurs with under-developed girls. The consequences are nervous disturbances. Because of the anaemia in these cases the red bone marrow is insufficiently supplied with blood-forming substances; above all, iron is lacking. Bodily growth is impaired, retarded.

Therefore the introduction of the aloe therapy in connection with the intake of iron is especially important in pediatrics.

The following therapy is recommended:

> To begin with, the patient is treated with ferruginous aloe syrup, i.e. syrupus aloes cum ferro.
> Aloe syrup is given at mealtimes, one teaspoon each three times a day. The treatment is continued for 12 days.
> In cases of more serious deficiency the doctor can prescribe an injection therapy after a treatment intermission, i.e. after the syrup cure. An interval of 20 days should be observed. After this, children receive a daily injection of 0,5 ml, adults of 1 ml, subcutaneously (thigh) for 15 days. Another intermission follows, this time of 30 days, whereupon the latter cure phase of 12 injections, same dosage as above, follows. This cure can be repeated after one year.

During the cure intermissions and after the treatment, adequate nutrition is of utmost importance. Here is some advice:

A great deal of ferruginous vegetables should be added to the diet. This includes spinach, sauerkraut, all leafy vegetables, stinging-nettle juice, plums, apricots, peaches; at least part of this vegetable and fruit diet should be eaten raw. All carriers of vitamin C are blood-forming. Therefore cherry juice, black currants, oranges, grapefruit and kiwi can also be recommended; moreover buttermilk and yoghurt. A change-over to whole-grain bread is also essential.

During their growing years, children should be given Silicea D 12 pills from biochemistry (two pills a day dissolved in the mouth), because this product promotes growth and cures the disturbances of the nails typical of anaemia.

The enclosed diagram demonstrates the enhancement of the blood-formation process after an aloe cure. It shows the result of a cure with aloe extract and makes visible the process of blood renewal after serious anaemia.

A — haemoglobin level in %
B — days of observation

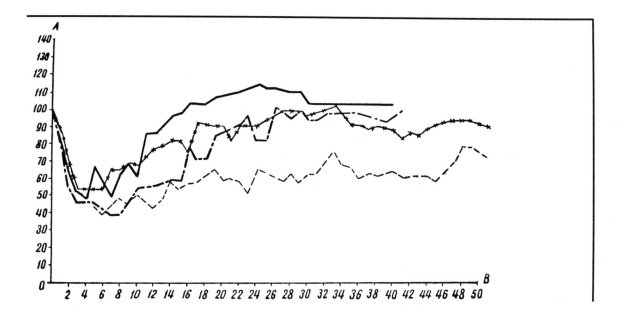

Before the cure: experiment —·—·—·—
                 control examination —————
After the cure: experiment _____
                 control examination x—x—x—x

ANILINISM

A veritable occupational disease with severe consequences. In combating this disease, so far all patients treated by doctors of Prof. Filatow's school have been completely cured.

Anilin poisoning with its late consequences should not be underestimated. It leads to asthma and allergies; it can also trigger cancer.

As the name says, this poisoning occurs with people working with anilin or its derivatives by breathing in the fumes.

Without realizing it, once can contract this affliction by frequently dyeing furs and leather articles. Symptoms are high blood pressure, irritability, disturbances in the gastro-intestinal tract.

The cure with aloe extract is to be administered as follows:

> **Either:** One ampulla containing 1 ml to be injected once a day under the skin (thigh), altogether 15 times, to be performed in the morning hours only!
>
> **Or:** Over a period of two weeks 20 to 30 minutes after lunch one teaspoon of aloe juice to be taken daily.

ARTERIOSCLEROSIS AND OTHER AGE-RELATED DISEASES

In general, academic medicine as well as practical experience are based on the belief that therapies to strengthen the body's defenses and to improve tonicity offer scant prospect of effecting advantageous changes at an advanced and high age. This may be true of conventional therapies, but it does not hold true for the aloe therapy.

Expressly because the confrontation of medical authorities in this country with this veritably revolutionizing therapy for geriatric diseases and cases of detrition has raised doubts, we will here report at great length about clinical experiences.

The human aging process is characterized by disturbances of the heart and circulation system. These disturbances are caused by processes of wear and decay as well as functional changes of the heart vessels, and through difficult changes in the regulation mechanisms which are responsible for a normal blood supply in the organs and tissue. In this way the symptoms of arteriosclerosis gradually develop. The tensions of the whole organism rise and, as a consequence, the elasticity of the vessel walls decreases. This lies at the bottom of the ever-increasing blood-circulation complaints. Because of impaired central regulation and increasing viscosity of the blood, wide-spread circulation problems occur. As we know, at an advanced age the reflexes weaken, in most cases also the supply of such hormones as insulin, cortisone and adrenalin is disturbed. Another impairment in the aging process involves the elasticity of the blood vessels. It is evident that all these impairments have a negative influence on the arterial pressure. At an advanced age, the functioning of the heart decreases, the rhythm of the heart contractions begins to become irregular, and the proportion between the working and the recreation phases of the heart deteriorates, i.e. the time of recreation decreases. All the above-mentioned developments cause oxygen deficiencies. According to various authors, up to 85% of the old people suffer from heart rhythm disturbances. The electrocardiograms show complicated biochemical aging processes of the nerve and muscle tissue of the heart, which become apparent in the changes of the electrical activity of the muscle apparatus of the heart, i.e. myocardium.

Therefore the geriatric investigations and research aim at combating the above-mentioned processes, and at preventive measures. Thus therapies must attack the causes for the disturbances within the heart and circulation system. Here the aloe therapy plays a central part. It promotes the normalization of impaired physiological processes within the sick organism; it increases the ability of regeneration and strengthens the body's own defenses. Thus aloe compounds have been successfully applied by different doctors in cases of degeneration. In all cases, the amount of cholesterol in the blood was noticeably lowered. Clinical observations of patients afflicted with arteriosclerosis of the vessels of the extremities confirmed after the aloe therapy a decrease of symptoms in all cases, with 30% of the patients even the disappearance of pains in the extremities. In many cases of arteriosclerosis treated with aloe, the patients' ability to work was restored. Medical doubts can be refuted with a complete documentation of the excellent results of the perennial clinical treatment of very old patients with aloe compounds.

Under the influence of the aloe therapy toward normalizing vasotonia, a beneficent change in the vessels of the eyes occurs. With 15 out of 46 older patients examined, an increased pressure within the central artery of the retina was noted, whereas the diameter of the vessel was almost normal. With ten of these patients the pressure within the central artery of the retina normalized after the aloe injections. This effect became even more pronounced after a repeated injection cure with aloe extract. The attending doctors were able to find that the normalization of vessel pressure in the eye was accompanied by normalizitation of blood pressure in general! An examination of the results of aloe cures makes evident that not only the circulatory system is normalized, but there are also effects on other functional systems of the organism, especially kidney function, which in its turn is in a close correlation with the activity of the heart and blood vessels. The doctors were able to note that the aloe therapies effect a noticeable stimulation of kidney function. This stimulating effect concerns the excreting functions of the kidneys as well as blood circulation within the kidneys. After the therapy, the blood supply of the kidneys is normalized. Moreover, an improved nitrogen elimination was confirmed. Here is an interesting comparison: in order to examine the effectiveness of the therapy, two age groups were assembled; one group of patients included people between 50 and 59, the other one between 60 and 74. The group of older patients experienced higher stimulation than the younger one. Both, however, noted long-lasting therapy success.

The active agents contained in the aloe, i.e. the biogenic stimulators, in their complicated biochemical structure resemble the biochemical structure of the organism; thus they fit into the subtle chemical structure of the cerebral enzyme systems, which effect the exchange of impulses between the central nervous system and the organs. Impulse exchange is understood to mean the information of the organs for the central nervous system concerning defects and deficiencies on the one hand, and the communication of orders from the central nervous system to the organs concerning the defense against, and elimination of, disturbances by mobilizing immune and healing mechanisms on the other hand.

The above-defined working mechanism explains the unusually broad pharmacological spectrum and the manifold influence on the function of virtually all organs and systems of the organism. It is because of the kinship of the biogenic stimulators from the aloe with the biochemical structures of the organism that they have a low toxicity and are almost free of side-effects.

The positive influence of the aloe therapy on improving the functions of kidneys and suprarenal glands normalizes the metabolic processes and eliminates a large number of symptoms which are caused by a poisoning of the organism through an imperfect metabolism.

Older people who have undergone the aloe therapy experience a long-lasting improvement of their general well-being. With about half the patients an improvement of vasotonia and heart functions was noted; a large majority confirmed a considerable improvement of varying degrees after one to four cures. These changes in the general well-being are derived from the considerable amelioration or the disappearance of many complaints which are so characteristic of senile decay. In summary the doctors report the following examples:

Spinal pains were cured, troubles and pains in the joints disappear, shortness of breath occurred less frequently, intestinal function was activated, dullness in the legs decreases, pounding of the heart and irregular heartbeat occur less frequently, dizziness disappears, sleeping normalizes to the point that barbiturates are no longer needed, so that the patient can be spared their troublesome side-effects. As a result of this therapy the mental activity and the ability to work increased, part of the patients regained their sexual prowess. It is a typical result of this therapy that older people experience renewed motivation and an increased interest in life. Therefore the aloe therapy can be strongly recommended for geriatrics, for the treatment of age-related ailments. This would have a humanizing effect on medical treatment and a considerable decrease of expenses of Public Health as long as the effects are correctly taken into account. Many patients who nowadays require continuous care and treatment in the hospital would be spared a hopeless condition if therapy were begun in time; in the case of inevitable aging processes they could be treated as out-patients while continuing their daily lives. In the long run, the aloe therapy means the preservation of a meaningful life for the individual, and an advantageous effect on the finances of Public Health.

Of course it should not be overlooked that the aloe therapy is successful in varying degrees: duration and constancy of successful cures vary; to a large extent they depend on the original state of health of the patient.

If for instance a patient paralyzed by a stroke is treated by the aloe therapy, the paralysis itself cannot be reversed. However, a strengthening of defenses and the mobilization of the will to survive can be effected. If on the other hand a patient shows the disposition or even symptoms of a stroke, such as the so-called »Schlägle« (i.e. minor stroke), which is seen as a precursor, a timely injection cure and aloe extract will prevent the stroke for a long time.

After the first, and even more so after the second injection cure, a positive effect can usually be observed. Third and fourth cures tend to be less effective. In the intervals between the cures the general well-being deteriorates, but rarely to the original stage.

In general it can be said that under the influence of aloe compounds the optimal effect of several enzymes is enhanced. The activity of the enzymes is stimulated. Tissue respiration as well as the activity of the enzyme systems within the heart tissue increase! Furthermore it was noted that aloe compounds increase the stimulation of reflexes and the responsiveness of the organism towards several medicaments, especially adrenalin, i.e. a characteristic stimulant of the sympathetic system. Dr. Arjajew, an eminent physician from the school of Prof. Filatow, formulates these findings as follows:

»The increase of the powers of adaptation and defense of the patient through the aloe therapy makes it possible to apply specifically directed medicaments to greater effect.«

Other doctors noted that an aloe-injection cure has a vasodilating effect and increases reaction reflexes of the central regulation apparatus of vasotonia; this effect on aging people cannot be over-estimated in the face of countless patients with angiosis and their considerable handicaps.

Even with very old patients a whole series of experimental observations has proven the stimulating influence of the aloe therapy on the function of the pancreas, the thyroid gland, and the suprarenal gland. The function of these endocrine glands is often seriously impaired at an advanced age.

It is especially the improved blood supply within human tissue that has a positive influence on the character and intensity of aging processes.

If the aloe therapy goes hand in hand with a reasonable diet with a balanced intake of vitamins and minerals, the general well-being of older people, and thus their vitality, can be positively influenced.

Experience has proved that with older people the dosage of the injection and the intervals between cures have to be adjusted on an individual basis. The doses for older people, especially for very old men, must be lower than for younger people. It is up to the doctor to determine the dosages individually.

It is now time to state the basic principles:

---

1. For patients up to 55 years of age:

The injections with aloe extract are applied for 30 days, once daily one ampulla of 1 ml, subcutaneously into the thigh. After that there is a phase of 30 days without injections. It is followed by the second part of the cure lasting again for 30 days: one injection a day as above.

2. For patients over 55:

Within a period of 50 days one ampulla of 0,5 ml of aloe extract is injected under the skin of the thigh every other day (altogehter 25 injections). An interval of 25 days of rest follows. The second phase of treatment with 15 injections continues with the following instructions: on the first three days one ampulla each of 0,5 ml is injected under the skin; from the fourth day on the above injections are administered ervery other day.

OINTMENT FOR ARTHRITIS

There are many kinds of arthritis, an inflammation of the joints, which in most cases is caused by disturbances in the uric acid level. The complaints occur in sudden attacks with indications of rheumatism of the joints. The attack is triggered by excitement, infection, colds, continuous state of nervousness, agitation and continuous nervous stress.

The following therapy is recommended:

Aloe ointment is to be rubbed lightly into the afflicted areas.

Food that is too rich should be avoided; no alcohol, no nicotine; lots of fresh fruit and vegetables, vegetable juices as well as birch juice from the pharmacy, health food store or drugstore three times a day — following the instructions on the package. Birch juice is especially effective in eliminating uric acid.

BRONCHIAL ASTHMA

A widespread disease of advanced civilization! Bronchial asthma — a neglected or chronic bronchitis quickly comes to mind! This applies to many cases. But it is not the whole truth! With many diseases we tend to neglect another cause: negative psychic experiences of our daily lives cause somatic illnesses. This can also be the case with bronchial asthma. In the same way that our psyche, general state of health and our genetic material condition us, diseases afflict us: a continuous state of excitement, anxiety, constant stress, discontent affect the organism at its weakest points. In one case this can be the stomach; here the inflammation of the gastromucous membrane can develop ulcers, duodenal ulcers may appear. In some cases it can be the bladder, or the nerves, in others acne, and among others it may be bronchial asthma.

This so-called neuropathic component is based on a high irritability of the personality. It is quite obvious that the therapy must be directed at the working mechanism of the central nervous system; for this purpose the aloe-extract cures with their specific effects are ideal. Many doctors have not recognized this neuropathic component of bronchial asthma; in many cases they treat only the symptoms, but not the root of the disease itself, and the complaints continue for the rest of the patient's life.

Of course there also exists the anatomic component, i.e. previous affliction with chronic bronchitis, or triggered by an allergy after the inhalation of dust, down, animal hair, fungi (mold) or chemical drugs, which cause the typical asthma attacks. Likewise the mental coming to terms with daily problems during attempted sleep can trigger the disease. If we consider how much all of us are exposed to such allergy-inducing factors because of ecological problems, that our children are imperiled at an early age by deteriorating ecological conditions, we must regard ourselves as lucky to have found a therapy which counteracts this tormenting disease. The acute attacks of asthma can trigger heart insufficiency, they considerably impair the patient's ability to work.

It has been proven that all aloe therapies have at least caused the disease to stagnate; repeated therapies have brought successful cures if the accompanying recommendations concerning nutrition and activity were observed and the mental causes were successfully tackled.

The following therapy is recommended:

---

1. On the first five days, one ampulla of 1 ml daily to be injected under the skin (thigh) in the morning hours. From the sixth through the fifteenth day, one injection of 1 ml is to be applied every day. An interval of 15 days follows. After that 20 more injections are given, one ampulla of 1 ml each every other day.

   After one year this cure is to be repeated.

With children afflicted with bronchial asthma caused by allergy or by croup or grippal croup, or croup resulting from measles and diphtheria, the following instructions apply:

On the first three days a daily injection of 0,5 ml is given under the skin (thigh); from the fourth through the fifteenth day an injection of 0,5 ml to be given every other day. After this there is an interval of ten days. During the following 30 days a total of 15 injections should be given, one every other day. A repetition after one year should not be necessary.

2. Lots of raw fruit and vegetables should be added to the diet, so that the membranes are strengthened through vitamins.

3. If the tonsils have not been removed they should be sucked clean and massaged.

4. Chest massages

5. Lungwort tea in the morning, at noon and in the evening with a spoonful of honey (preferably thyme or eucalyptus honey)

6. Little or no alcohol, no nicotine

7. The patient's self-assurance must be psychologically invigorated. The person afflicted with bronchial asthma tends to be discouraged and to have serious difficulties of adaptation. Therefore his self-assurance needs to be strengthened; he must be given the chance to relax and to talk about his problems in an atmosphere of trust.

EYE DISEASES

EGYPTIAN OPHTHALMIA

Scientifically called trachoma or trachomatous conjunctivitis, this disease must be reported to the authorities. »Egyptian ophthalmia« is an infectious, extraordinarily intractable, sometimes chronic form of conjunctivitis which ought to be taken seriously.

At the early stage with its formation of follicular growths, trachoma granulations (trachoma from ancient Greek for »rough«); later an infection of the tarsus and gelatinous swelling; in its late stage formation of scar tissue, accompanied by contraction of the conjunctiva. Almost every chronic trachoma eventually spreads to the cornea. Every trachoma can lead to blindness.

Now at long last a natural remedy for this dangerous affliction has been found.

The subcutaneous injections of the aloe extract are to be applied as follows:

The compound, a watery solution in ampullas of 1 ml each for adults is best injected once a day in the evening under the skin of the thigh, i.e. not into the vein or muscle, but subcutaneously, technically comparable to the injections of diabetics. A series of 30 injections is recommended. In case the disease should not have disappeared completely, after an interval of 30 days another series of 30 injections, 1 ml daily, should be given.

Children of five years or older receive injections of 0,5 ml, one every other day, until 16 − 20 injections have been reached. If the child's ailment should turn out to be persistent, after an interval of 30 days a second injection phase can be administered, with the same rhythm as the first one. − During the treatment an eye ablution with camomile tea or fennel tea is recommended. Utmost cleanliness must be observed.

CHOROIDITIS

Choroiditis is an inflammation of the choroid membrane. The inflammation becomes visible in the fundus of the eye. In most cases it is accompanied by retinitis. It is often caused by an infection (toxoplasmosis) contracted by eating infected meat, raw eggs, or from acutely infected pets.

A proven therapy is the same that is given in the chapter on advanced myopia.

BLEPHARITIS

This disease, an inflammation of the eyelids, occurs frequently. In general, blepharitis is seen as a seborrhea of the eyes (pathological changes in the secretion of the sebaceous glands). Faulty refraction of the light can be the cause. − The symptoms are itching, redness and slight swelling of the rims of the eyelids. It often starts out with tiny flakes of skin at the base of the eyelashes. If not treated, small abscesses and festering ulcers may appear. Therefore the dandruff on the eyelashes should not be overlooked as a minor blemish!

Recommended therapy for grown-ups:

An aloe emulsion (emulsum aloes, cf. special section) to be rubbed gently into the infected eyelids twice a day − mornings and evenings. In case of more acute indications an injection cure with aloe extract is advisable as follows:

During the first nine days one injection to be given every other day; on the following nine days one injection of 1 ml of aloe extract daily (i.e. altogehter 14 injections in 18 days).

By then the treatment should have been successful.

As the aloe extract strengthens the eye nerves and increases vision − the author has been able to verify reports that even patients over 70 have experienced and increase of vision from 60 to 90% − a cure with aloe extract besides its specific healing properties effects a general strengthening of the central nervous system and an organic invigoration. Nevertheless the **therapy instructions must be strictly observed, because an overdose**, same as in other cases, **has harmful effects**. After completion of the first phase, there is an interval of 30 days. Afterwards a second series consisting of 15 injections follows at the same interval as in the first series.

The therapy should be complemented by a raw-food diet, mainly grapefruit, which lower the blood pressure. Another useful complement is kiwi and papaya, a kind of melon; moreover garlic pills, which are available in health food stores and pharmacies.

CONJUNCTIVITIS (PINK-EYE)

This is an inflammation of the conjunctiva. We can differentiate between the acute simple conjunctivitis, i.e. conjunctival catarrh, and chronic conjunctivitis. With the acute catarrh, the symptom is vehement reddening and swelling together with profuse excretions. With a chronic inflammation, however, there is no papilledema; the excretions are less profuse. According to Römer, the excrescence of the papilla of the optic nerve gives the diseased area the looks of shorn velvet.

Acute conjunctivitis is caused by dust, draft, cold, foreign matter entering the eye, smoke.

At the basis of conjunctivitis we find a poor general condition of the patient with an inclination toward catarrhs, chronically cold feet, the wearing of spectacles whose lenses are no longer adequate, chronic inflammation of nasal membranes as well as dacryocystectasia. The disease is triggered in the same way as acute conjunctival catarrh.

With children we know a special kind of disease afflicting the conjunctiva, i.e. spring conjunctivitis, which ought to be taken seriously, because if it is neglected or treated inadequately it can become chronic.

Besides, there is one variety of the disease on a tubercular basis: nodulous concunctivitis. It is traced back to glandular tuberculosis. In this case, limp festering ulcers form in the conjunctiva with a coating as white as curds. As a consequence the conjunctiva may contract.

The following cure with aloe extract is to be used against all kinds of conjunctivitis:

---

1. Simple conjunctivitis, conjunctival catarrh with adults

The extract, in ampullas of 1 ml each, is injected subcutaneously into the thigh every other day, once in the morning or evening. 15 injections normally suffice. During and after the disease, eye ablutions with fennel or camomile tea can be recommended over a period of time. The author prefers fennel.

2. Chronic conjunctivitis with adults

We recommend the injection of 1 ml under the skin of the thigh once a day, in the morning or evening, altogether 16 times.

If this treatment is successful it should be terminated. In stubbornly chronic cases, after an interval of 30 days a second cure phase with another 16 injections can follow.

3. Nodulous conjunctivitis with adults

Here the injection cure with aloe extract lasts 30 days: during the first phase of treatment 1 ml a day is to be injected before bedtime. After an interval of 30 days the second cure phase of 30 injections, daily one ampulla of 1 ml each, follows. In most cases the cause of the tubercular origin will thus be eliminated. As the aloe extract through its working mechanism via the central nervous system invigorates the defenses of the patient's body, the immune system is especially strengthened against such diseases. As a complementary therapy and for after-treatment, sun baths for the whole body (no solariums!) are important.

4. Conjunctivitis with children

In most cases a cure of 15 injections of 0,5 ml applied subcutaneously into the thigh will suffice. The injections should be given every other evening before bedtime, so that after 30 days the treatment is completed. Only to be used for children **over five years of age**.

Especially in the case of children, daily ablutions with fennel tea are recommended, with the tea being nice and warm.

FUCHS'S ATROPHY

This eye affliction is very unpleasant. It is a black spot in the macula, and develops through myopia on account of mechanical changes, i.e. with dilation atrophy (weakness), with lacerations as well as bleeding.

As a consequence, central vision is considerably diminished. In severe cases total blindness can set in. The disease was named after the Viennese oculist Ernst Fuchs (1851 – 1930).

Especially with older patients, ophthalmology has no cure to offer.

In 1983 a 72-year-old woman consulted the author in Berlin; through her life companion she had heard about the aloe research done by the ARBEITSGEMEINSCHAFT GRUNDLAGENFORSCHUNG FÜR BIOLOGISCHE MEDIZIN, and she knew that one field of this research was ophthalmology. Moreover she had heard that veritable floods of pilgrims from all over the world were streaming to the institute of Prof. Filatow in Odessa for the cure of their eye disease for which Western academic medicine does not know any therapies.

The researchers wanted to help this woman. Her central vision was so diminished that she placed dishes, for instance, beside the table; regardless of such unpleasant consequences of the disease, impaired vision of this kind causes a continuous nervous stress, which at an advanced age the immune powers are not able to cope with. If, however, the body's defenses are further weakened, blindness of the afflicted eye may set in.

At the time, the patient was being treated by a competent oculist, who was at a loss herself and sent her to an internationally renowned specialist in the field of academic medicine. This specialist in his turn had no therapy. When the patient alluded to Prof. Filatow and new findings, the ophthalmic surgeon indicated with regret that he was not able to help. He had worked with Filatow and respected the famous oculist, but he did not know that in the meantime the German group had successfully proved the effect of the aloe therapy. With patients over 60 he did not see a therapy with any prospect of success, and he handed the material back to the patient without treating her. He too confirmed the Fuchs's atrophy, which the oculist had correctly diagnosed before; the diagnosis was correct, but for the patient that was to no avail.

Based on the experience available to the scientists in Berlin she decided to help herself with the biostimulated aloe extract. She was in despair about her disease and the resulting impairment of her life, but she did not give up hope. She is a rational personality, energetic, with executive experience, who had mastered other ailments before. She applied the aloe injections herself as follows:

For 30 days one daily injection of 1 ml each subcutaneously (under the skin of the thigh) in the morning hours, followed by a short rest. After this first phase of thirty days there was an interval of another 30 days. Thereupon the second cure phase of 30 daily injections of 1 ml each in the morning hours followed.

The results turned out to be a great surprise:

First day: worsening of condition; black spot grew in size
Second day: almost unchanged worsening of condition
Third day: Fuchs's atrophy shifts
From the fourth day on: slow dissolution of the shadowy spot, which by the thirtieth day does not return.

As another consequence, continuous improvement of vision and of the general condition was noted. After the end of the first cure phase of 30 days, i.e. during the interval of rest, the spot returned intermittently for short periods during the morning hours. After the completion of the second cure phase of 30 days it disappeared completely, and by publication date, i.e. almost two years after the cure, it has not reappeared. It is noteworthy that the patient's vision, who at the time was 72, had increased by the end of the cure from 60 % to 90 %.

Six months after the end of the therapy a slight age-related deterioration of vision occurred, but it has to be noted that the habitually active patient put herself under great strain in her large household; in other words, she did not take proper care of herself, which would have been advisable.

This experience demonstrates that in case of an advanced aging process with its wear and decay, the therapy should be repeated after a year. This can be done up to four times in the following years.

About one year after the first cure the patient decided upon a second one. Her general condition improved and she was able to retain her vision at the previous level. The most important result however was that the Fuchs's atrophy, this irritating, dangerous black shadow, did not reappear. The patient is now cured, and she does not need to undergo expensive treatment in Odessa.

GRAY CATARACT

The gray cataract is an increasing clouding of the lens. Usually this clouding does not occur before the 60th year of age. It starts out on the rim and eventually covers the whole lens. This causes deteriorating vision, which becomes increasingly blurred. Finally the afflicted person is unable to distinguish between light and dark.

The fact that this affliction sets in at an advanced age makes evident that its cause is to be found in a general weakness, the diminishing of the strength of the nerves, above all a lack of pro-vitamin A and C, in many cases also a consequence of life-long onesided nutrition. Other causes can be diabetes, eye injuries and innate cloudiness.

The aloe-extract therapy will be able at any rate to arrest the disease; it will strengthen the body's defenses, revitalize and invigorate the eye nerves and preserve the patient's vision. This amounts to a great deal. Thus an injection cure should be worthwhile in this case too. The instructions are as follows:

For 30 days one ampulla of 1 ml each is to be injected subcutaneously into the thigh. Afterwards the usual interval of 30 days should be observed. Subsequently another daily injection for 30 days. At the same time the diet should become low in salt! The intake of vitamins C and A is essential. This applies to all kinds of citrus fruit and kiwi, carrot juice and raw carrots grown biologically (health food store). The frequent intake of tomatoes is an ideal complement of the orange, kiwi and grapefruit diet. The aloe cure should be started as soon as the first signs of impaired vision occur between 40 and 50, the harbingers of gray cataract. With the cure being repeated up to three times, i.e. a span of four years, and changing nutrition to a preponderantly vegetarian diet, the development of gray cataract can be completely prevented.

An operation will not be the ideal solution. After all it effects only a partial restoration of vision with the help of the well-known cataract spectacles.

The apostle Thomas is reported, before he went on his mission to India, to have taken over a method of Arabic medicine on the Yemenitic isle of Sokotra, to heal cataracts with the fresh juice of the Sokotra aloe growing there, one of the most valuable plants of the aloe family. He restored the vision of many old people, later on in India too.

GREEN CATARACT

Green and gray cataracts are two diseases with entirely different causes. The green cataract — science calls it glaucoma — is caused by an abnormal increase of pressure inside the eye. As a consequence, optic nerve and retina are seriously damaged. The disease can lead to total blindness. It is important to pay attention to the early warning signs of the green cataract. Here are some important symptoms:

Seeing spectral colors, all objects are seen as if through a smoky haze, or the patient thinks he must look through a wall of mist, the reaction to light becomes sluggish, the pupils widen. The acute phase is characterized by disturbances of vision, the field of vision is concentrically restricted. With rising pressure, excruciating pain sets in, which extends throughout the head and is often accompanied by nausea and vomiting. The deterioration of vision increases to the point when light and dark can no longer be distinguished. At an advanced stage the disease comes in sudden seizures. The causes may be found in other eye diseases, such as iritis, phacometachoresis, irritation of the ciliary zonule, tumors of the eyeball etc., or a nervous disease.

Now the oculist can be provided with a means which effects a considerable improvement of the disease and a complete cure without an operation.

The aloe-extract cure is to be applied as follows:

> Duration of the complete cure for adults: three months.
>
> During the first phase 1 ml of the extract is injected daily into the thigh on 30 consecutive days. An interval of 30 days without injections follows. After this another series of injections (30 injections of 1 ml each daily over a period of 30 days).
>
> After one year this cure is to be repeated. In the first year the disease is favorably influenced and arrested, in the second year it will be completely cured.

With this serious eye disease it is of utmost importance to keep a diet low in salt, containing plenty of fruit and raw food. Intake of liquid should be restricted. Veritable thirst cures are helpful until the pressure has normalized. During acute attacks of glaucoma the patient must stay in bed. The eye has to be cooled. The green cataract has derived its name from a greenish tinge of the pupil — instead of black.

Aloe-extract injection therapy with GREEN CATARACT (GLAUCOMA)

a) before treatment b) after 11 injections c) after 35 injections

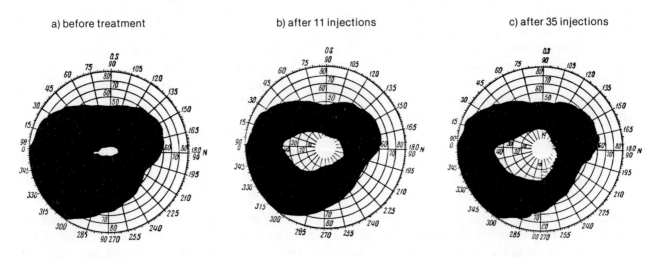

The pictures show the changes of the field of vision of a glaucoma patient before and after aloe treatment
The widespread shadowing of the field of vision is in this case decisively reduced after a short period of treatment!

KERATITIS

There are many kinds of corneal ailments. For all of them therapies have now become available in the West which in the eye clinic of Odessa, named after the oculist Prof. Filatow, have effected remarkable and constant cures after passing rigorous clinical tests.

Keratitis fasciculosa, a kind of corneal inflammation, tends to be seriously understimated; it is triggered by metabolic disturbances on the surface of the cornea, and it is recognized by the development of tiny calcium laminae.

The inflammation of deeper layers of the cornea often has a tubercular cause. In most cases, however, the disease can be traced back to innate syphilis.

A widerspread variety is the inflammatory clouding of the corneal surface. It can have various causes: Neglected conjunctivitis, tuberculosis, scrofulosis and, last but not least, injuries.

The symptoms are constant watering, sensitivity to light, blood-vessel growths.

Frequently to be observed: the blister-shaped corneal inflammation on the surface. It is also known by the name Herpes corneae.

The process is long and tedious. Corneal ulcers may develop. The inflammation leads to the formation of tiny blisters which are interconnected by a fissure.

Recently, keratitis has frequently developed following a virus infection. Also after a trauma keratitis may develop. The so-called keratitis electrica is a typical variety of civilization. It is caused by ultraviolet radiation, which damages the cornea, e.g. after electro-welding without goggles. Corneal damage, which is very dangerous and, unfortunately, very widerspread, can be traced back to artificial sunlight (solarium). In this case instructions are often foolishly neglected.

Corneal ulcers may also develop. In most cases they appear after the loss of tissue on the surface of the cornea. They can also be caused by injuries of the cornea (e.g. grain stalks, twigs etc.), as well as invading bacteria, which cause loss of tissue. In many cases the iris is likewise inflamed, which then clogs the front of the lens. In most cases there is the danger of corneal rupture. Another consequence can be the suppuration of the eyeball. An especially negative aspect is that corneal ulcers leave scars.

According to the author, the clouding of the cornea should be named »white cataract«. This comes closest to its importance, its development and its consequences.

The successful cures with aloe extract have been constant in all cases of keratitis.

These are the instructions concerning therapy:

1. Corneal inflammations of all kinds

On 22 days one ampulla daily of 1 ml each of aloe extract to be injected under the skin, either in the morning or evening. After an interval of 15 days, the second cure phase comprising 15 ampullas of 1 ml each follows, to be applied daily, one injection in the morning or evening.

Children are given injections of 0,5 ml each every other day in late afternoon; altogether 15 injections, so that the cure is completed after 30 days. In persistent cases an interval of rest of 30 days is to be observed, followed by a second cure phase of another 15 injections, spread over 30 days, i.e. every other day an injection of 0,5 ml.

As in all pediatric therapies, only children over five years of age may be treated with aloe injections!

Aloe treatment of keratitis with formation of blisters

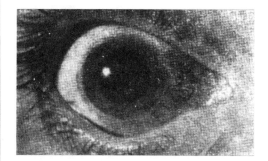 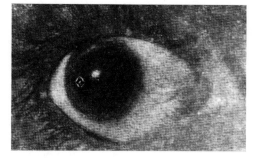

Before treatment with aloe-extract injection   after treatment

2. Corneal ulcers

In this case the disease is usually more persistent; therefore a cure of 30 days, i.e. one injection daily in the morning or evening is recommended for adults. After an interval of 30 days another cure phase follows, with 30 ampullas of 1 ml each to be injected into the thigh at the rate of one injection daily.

With adults the cure can be repeated after one year if necessary.

The author suggests mornings or evenings as the time of application if no other prescription exists. Patients with high blood pressure are advised to apply the injections only in the morning or afternoon, because they have a slight stimulating effect.

If children five years of age or older suffer from corneal ulcers the oculist should conduct an injection cure of 44 days, injecting one ampulla of 0,5 ml every other day (altogether 22 injections). After a pause of 30 days the second cure phase with another 22 injections in 44 days (one injection every other day) follows.

With the above-mentioned eye diseases, keeping a raw-food diet is of vital importance. With all eye afflictions, a vegetarian diet low in salt is advisable. We especially recommend fresh juice available in pharmacies, health food stores, drug stores etc., biologically grown vegetables, above all carrot juice, vegetable juice, cherry juice. Furthermore we recommend getting plenty of fresh air, especially at the seashore, because of the iodine in the air.

Accompanying therapies such as after-treatment are also of great importance for the healing process. This includes eye ablutions with warm fennel tea, putting moist, hot bags of camomile on the eyes, and immediately afterwards moist, cool water compresses. These ribbon-like compresses are placed over both eyes and temples. This therapy has been very successfully used by the great naturopath Dr. Brauchle. The author can testify that these remedies complement the aloe cure most effectively. Not to be forgotten, whenever possible, are sun baths, with the eyes being well protected!

MYOPIA

Myopia is a widespread phenomenon.

We can distinguish between benign myopia and indications of a malignant variety. In many cases diabetes is the cause, sometimes it is the side-effect of chemical medicaments. Myopia is characterized by the fact that parallel rays converge in front of the iris, because the fraction of light within the eye is too strong or the eyeball is too slow (definition according to Pschyrembel).

Youthful myopia, which is regarded as benign, stops at puberty. Progressive myopia, however, causes an alteration of the eyeground, which is not to be found in the first variety. Degeneration of the choroid membrane sets in.

Instructions for therapy:

---

1. Benign myopia

On 15 consecutive days one ampulla of aloe extract of 0,5 ml each is injected subcutaneously. After a pause of 15 days, the second phase of treatment with 15 ampullas of 0,5 ml each, spread over 15 days, follows.

2. Progressive myopia

On 15 consecutive days one ampulla of aloe extract of 1 ml each is injected subcutaneously. After a pause of another 15 days the second phase of treatment with 1 ml each on 30 consecutive days follows.

After one year the cure should be repeated.

RETINITIS

The term retinitis comprises various ailments afflicting the retina: the inflammation of the choroid membrane is accompanied by opacity of the vitreous body, occasionally also by retinopexy. The basic cause is often the process of degeneration. Sometimes the disease is also triggered by measles.

In the course of the disease the nerve elements of the retina go under and bone-corpuscle-like pigments are deposited. The disease progresses from the periphery toward the center. The characteristic symptom is a restriction of vision. Retinitis pigmentosa can lead to blindness. Classic retinitis usually means a serous inflammation which also afflicts the choroid membrane covering the retina. Numerous little hemorrhages develop in the retina, accompanied by general or local circulation disturbances. Hypertension, i.e. high blood pressure, can have an extremely negative influence on the disease.

Therefore it is necessary to combine the aloe-extract therapy with the intake of whitethorn juice, fresh juice from the health food store or drops from the pharmacy. Whereas the application of aloe may slightly raise the blood pressure of certain patients, pure whitethorn juice effects a normalizing of the blood pressure, so that no counter-indications or side-effects appear.

Therapy instructions for retinitis with adults:

1. With the whitethorn drops the dosage prescribed in the instructions must be strictly obeyed: they should be taken twice a day: for the first time after breakfast, for the second time before going to bed. Contrary to instructions, which recommend dilution, fresh juice is to be taken undiluted after meals in the morning and evening, 1 tablespoon each.

2. Over a period of 30 days the aloe extract is injected under the skin (thigh), every other day 1 ml each. The injections should be administered in late afternoon only (4:00 – 6:00 P.M.).

ATROPHY OF THE OPTIC NERVE

The disease is better known under its Latin term: atrophia nervi optici. An atrophy can be defined as the weakness of an organ, with number and size of cells decreasing.

Causes often are nutritional and metabolic disturbances.

But also cerebral and spinal ailments can trigger this weakness. It can also be hereditary. Other frequent causes can be inflammations of the nerves, or various protracted eye afflictions. Also traumatic connections have been noted.

We can distinguish between total and partial atrophy. In both cases the therapy with aloe extract brings about lasting cures. It strengthens the cells. The following instructions apply:

For a period of 15 days 1 ml of aloe extract to be injected daily under the skin of the thigh. After a 14-day interval, another cure with one injection daily follows. After half a year this cure is to be repeated with the same interval, and one year after this to be repeated again.

By then the atrophy will have disappeared; number and size of the cells function adequately.

Also in this case a change of diet with special emphasis on a vegetarian diet, preferably fruit with plenty of vitamin C, and vegetables with plenty of vitamin A, such as carrots, is important.

More and more often children are afflicted by such an atrophy.

Instructions for children:

Children five years of age or older are given one injection of 0,5 ml of aloe extract under the skin of the thigh every other day for 15 times, so that the first cure phase lasts 30 days. After an interval of 30 days, one ampulla of 0,5 ml each is injected daily for 14 consecutive days.

Providing the children with vitamins C and A is of utmost importance.

ALOE AS EYE PROTECTION

The chapters on ophthalmology demonstrate the versatility of aloe compounds. As the biogenic stimulators of the aloe extract – through their working mechanism via the central nervous system – mainly improve vision, even healthy people should make use of the protective powers of the aloe to secure this state of health. This pertains especially to deterioration of vision.

Clinical experiments have shown that the aloe therapy not only normalizes vasotonia, but also works favorable changes in the vessels of the eyes. Among 40 elderly patients examined, 15 had increased pressure in the central artery of the retina, whereas the diameter of the artery was almost normal. In ten of these patients the pressure within the central artery of the retina normalized after aloe injections. The normalization of vessel pressure in the eye was accompanied by normalization of blood pressure in general.

The following instructions are recommended:

> Once a week 1 ml of aloe extract is to be injected subcutaneously into the thigh. The duration of this cure is six months. For children five years or older, use 0,5 ml per injection, otherwise same procedure.
>
> For the diet it is important that food containing plenty of pro-vitamin A, above all carrot juice, be taken. Other foods rich in pro-vitamin A, which in the organism turns into vitamin A, are apricots, tomatoes, rose hips, celery, spinach, cabbage and stinging nettle. Foods richest in vitamin A are cod liver oil, butter and milk.

RHEUMATOID SPONDYLITIS

This is a widespread illness which usually appears in the third decade of life. The Latin name, morbus Bechterew, is derived from the Russian doctor and psychologist Vladimir Bechterew, who worked with Wilhelm Wundt in Leipzig, and with Charcot in Paris, among others. In a way rheumatoid spondylitis starts out treacherously, because in its early stages, at a time when academic medicine would have to offer promising therapies, it is usually not recognized. The pains tend to be diagnosed as rheumatic inflammations. Therefore in case of complaints resembling rheumatism the patient is well advised to undergo immediate X-ray examinations, especially in the area of the sacrum. This disease is of immense social importance, because it can lead to the inability to work and to permanent invalidity.

The disease is an inflammation of the bone-joint system. The cause is as yet unknown. The author suspects metabolic disturbances. It is a noteworthy fact that men rather than women are afflicted. In the course of this ailment the swivel joints become inflamed and ossify until they become completely rigid. At the same time the costovertebral joints are afflicted. The disease progresses in spurts, when the stiffening spine worsens from spurt to spurt under almost unbearable pain. Only after complete rigidness, i.e. at the end of the process, does the pain subside: by then the spinal column is completely immobile. During the latter stages, breathing disorders and changes in the lungs occur.

The following therapy is recommended:

> 1. The diet should be changed, same as with rheumatic diseases, to foods low in salt, mainly a raw-fruit and vegetable diet.
> 2. Hot sand and sun baths
> 3. Remedial gymnastics, especially swimming
> 4. Massages, if possible daily, so as to preserve the degenerating muscle tissue of the back
> 5. Injection cure with aloe extract as follows:
>
>   Over a period of 30 days one ml of aloe extract to be injected subcutaneously into the thigh every morning, to be followed by 15 to 20 minutes of rest. After an interval of 30 days the second cure phase sets in with another 30 injections, 1 ml each daily.
>
>   After one year the cure is to be repeated.

EPILEPSY

The historical fact that during the battle of Leipzig Napoleon suffered an epileptic seizure points out that this is a neurologic affliction. For the first time it usually appears between the onset of puberty and the 20th year of age. The causes are still not completely clear, but there are some indications:

metabolic poisoning, head and brain injuries, cerebral growths, but also hysteria lead to spasmodic seizures with loss of consciousness, screaming — followed by deep exhaustion. These are indications of traumatic epilepsy. But there is also a hereditary epilepsy, which can be caused by alcoholism of a parent, but also by syphilis. Characteristically the epileptic wants to move around: he runs quickly, his steps seem restless and hurried. When we think of the Bible's »punishments« reaching into future generations, we are beginning to grasp the meaning: it is not the act of punishment as such that we are warned against, but the fact that cardinal sins against our health have inescapable consequences, which by genetic law we pass on to our children and grandchildren. That this can be punishment too is demonstrated most emphatically by this disease.

With the aloe-injection therapy the neurologist is given a biological means of therapy which positively influences the course of the disease. An experienced neurologist will make sure that the psychological treatment of the patient will increase his hope to the point of conviction that his ailment can improve considerably and that his seizures will appear with decreasing frequency. Prof. Meljanko from Kiev reports successful cures of epilepsy.

Prof. Rosenzweig stresses the fact that the aloe-extract cure has a stimulating effect on the whole organism and strengthens its defenses. At the same time the other specifically directed methods of treatment are made more effective.

According to Prof. Rosenzweig the main salutary effect of the aloe therapy is its anticonvulsive influence in cases of post-traumatic epilepsy (i.e. after injuries). The spastic seizures occurred less frequently and after several cures ceased completely! Other physicians confirmed this report in cases of craniocerebral traumas. Likewise, Dr. Ulit among others confirmed in the case of cerebral circulatory disturbances that after aloe-extract injections the motoric functions improved and speech was restored.

WOMEN'S DISEASES

Menstrual complaints, such as the failure to appear, delayed or excessive menstruation are among the tormentors of the female population. Abdominal inflammations have various causes and appear in many different forms. The most protracted kind are the festering abdominal ailments. Now, for all of them, a thorough and harmless therapy without any side-effects has been found. This is especially important for women's diseases, as there is a strong tendency towards recurrence and relapse. Here again the invigoration of the body's defenses is the uppermost principle. In combination with a natural life style, an aloe-extract therapy eliminates the causes of the disease reliably and in a biological manner.

Instructions are as follows:

In case of menstrual disturbances, every other day an injection of 0,5 ml is administered subcutaneously into the thigh. Altogehter 15 injections of this kind are given.

After three months the second cure follows; after another three months the treatment is to be repeated as above.

For festering abdominal ailments the following therapy is recommended:

One daily injection of 1 ml of aloe extract into the thigh for 30 consecutive days **with the exception of the days of the monthly period.** (Injectios are to be stopped from the day before the period sets in through one day after the period is over!) After this an interval of 30 injection-free days is to be observed. It is followed by the second cure phase with another 30 injections (mind the menstruation pause again!).

In addition, patients are recommended to drink Lady's Mantle tea once or twice a day, and on some days to observe a raw-fruit and vegetable diet. Agave juice as well as cherry and birch juice enhance the blood-cleansing process.

GASTRITIS

Gastritis is an inflammation of the gastric membranes; it is a widespread and growing civilized ailment. In its acute form, this disease is caused by deficient nutrition: food eaten too hot, drinks taken too cold, »gobbling« down food, insufficient chewing, excessive intake of coffee, alcohol and nicotine are the causes of membranal irritations, which precede gastritis. A typical symptom is the feeling of fullness: after initial appetite, stomach pains and headache set in together with eructation. The stomatic flora changes disagreeably; halitosis often is the precursor of poor stomach conditions and membranal ailments.

Quite often, however, gastritis is a nervous side-effect of constant stress; the person pressured by deadlines and haunted by existential anxieties is predestined for chronic gastritis. As the course of this disease can be protracted and rarely stops unless the patient forgoes toxic stimulants or heavy food, we recommend the following aloe treatment to bring about an early amelioration, and finally a full cure.

In the case of acute gastritis the following therapy should be observed: take one teaspoon of bio-stimulated aloe juice – succus aloes – two or three times a day after meals. The cure should last between three weeks and two months.

In serious cases, i.e. if the disease lasts for more than two months, as well as in the case of chronic gastritis, an injection cure with aloe extract is required as follows:

For 15 consecutive days one injection of aloe extract to be administered subcutaneously (thigh) in the morning hours; after an injection-free interval of 20 days, 15 more injections follow as above, 1 ml each. During the injection phase no aloe juice is to be taken, because over-medication may have harmful effects.

It is essential to change over to a raw-fruit and vegetable diet, muesli, steamed potatoes in their skins with cottage cheese (without linseed oil), crisp bread. Later, as healing progresses, moderate portions of meat, fish or scrambled eggs can be added.

INFLAMMATION OF THE AUDITORY NERVE (HARDNESS OF HEARING)

The so-called neuritis acustica is an inflammation of the nervus acusticus. It appears in the form of hardness of hearing in both ears, buzzing in the ears, the feeling of pressure in both ears, various ear noises, and disturbances of equilibrium.

It can be caused by damages through chemical drugs, e.g. quinine, salicylic acid, as well as poisoning through alcohol, lead and bacteria. Among further causes we often find neglected typhoid and scarlet fever as well as diphtheria. A woman doctor was consulted by a patient of advanced age who was suffering from hardness of hearing and buzzing in the ears. Her previous doctor had tried to convince her that her ailment was a consequence of arteriosclerosis, to be accepted as an effect of her years. The doctor made a more thorough analysis, found out that years before a scarlet-fever infection had been neglected, and prescribed an injection cure with bio-stimulated aloe extract. After two cures the patient was able to hear normally. We must add, however, that during the cure she was put on a preponderantly vegetarian diet. Forgoing toxic stimulants of all kinds is important.

In the case of inflammation of the auditory nerve the following therapy is recommended:

Three times a week 1 ml of aloe extract is to be injected subcutaneously under the skin of the thigh. After 18 injections an interval of 30 days is to be observed, to be followed by another cure phase with another three injections of 1 ml each a week, until 24 injections have been given. Altogether the cure comprises 42 injections.

LOSS OF HAIR

Another term for this affliction is alopecia.

In case of mental causes an aloe cure can be helpful. To determine whether loss of hair has psychic causes, the personality of the patient must be closely analyzed.

It is always a certain type of personality that tends toward, or suffers from, phobias. There are many variations: phobias of all kinds are mostly unfounded anxieties. The feeling of fear forces the patient to commit certain acts, or to forgo them; There is the fear of crossing open spaces, fear of bridges (the patient is afraid of falling if he looks over the railing), the fear of using elevators and escalators, as well as intellectual and psychic inadequacy, i.e. not being able to cope with one's professional demands. It is always a case of continuous stress or hysteria. Excessive fear of cancer belongs here too.

Hawaiians report among other things that rubbing aloe juice into the scalp is supposed to arrest loss of hair. To make one thing quite clear, however: as yet a remedy for loss of hair has not been found. Thus neither aloe juice nor extract is such a remedy. In case of psychic causes of alopecia, however, an injection cure with aloe extract can arrest the loss of hair. And that should be a good enough result: retaining whatever hair is left.

The aloe-extract cure is to be applied as follows:

For 30 consecutive days one ampulla of 1 ml to be injected under the skin (thigh); afterwards an interval of 30 days without injections is to be observed, to be followed by another cure phase of 30 days, one injection of 1 ml daily. At the same time, burdock oil should be rubbed into the scalp: head massages as well as ultra-violet sunray treatment are recommended. Little or no alcohol!

In case of achronic pelada (hair falls out in circles), the afflicted areas should be rubbed with soft medicinal soap from the pharmacy.

HAEMORRHOIDS

Haemorrhoids can be defined as widenings and protrusions of veins outside and inside the anus. Frequent causes are constipation, lack of movement, especially in the case of a sedentary life style, as well as inflammations of abdominal organs, liver ailments and heart diseases. One frequently overlooked, but common cause is chronically cold feet. When the haemorrhoidal knots are irritated, they cause violent itching or stinging pain, the anus is no longer tight, mucus and liquid intestinal contents ooze out. Through fissures the skin begins to change. Hard stool scratches the haemorrhoids open, so that they start bleeding. As a consequence, intestinal membranes are damaged, ulcers and festering wounds form in the anus.

As a first priority, regular and light stool must be provided for. Part of this is guaranteed by healthy nutrition rich in bulkage. Also a tea therapy helps to make digestion function properly and to produce soft stools. The tea should be mixed from one part each of dried aloe leaves (bio-stimulated), one part of ortosiphonis, and one part of Tinnevelly-Sennes fruit. One moderately heaped teaspoon of the above mixture per cup suffices; one cup in the evening is enough. This serves as a basis for a supportive therapy with aloe extract. The aloe extract eliminates above all the congestion of the venous flow of blood, and it invigorates liver and heart.

Once a week 1 ml of bio-stimulated extract is injected subcutaneously into the thigh. The cure lasts for three months.

For treating the afflicted skin we recommend a hot rinsing of the anus, to be followed by dabbing with olive oil. If this treatment is not successful, hamamelis ointment should be rubbed in. After completion of the aloe injection cure 8 – 10 drops of the medicament Paeonia Oligoplex should be diluted in water in a liqueur glass and taken three times a day. This treatment lasts for four weeks; if necessary it can be prolonged. If so, the doctor should be consulted. Full baths with horse-chestnut blossoms are recommended as a complementary therapy.

CUTANEOUS TUBERCULOSIS

The great number of different varieties of cutaneous tuberculosis are grouped together under the scientific name tuberculosis cutis. One of the most frequent varieties is lupus vulgaris. Tiny nodes appear in the skin, mainly in the face, in the cheeks and at the root of the nose. Gradually they spread and eventually infect almost all of the healthy skin. This is a case of tubercular bacilli with the body being otherwise free of tuberculosis.

Another variety of this disease appears with increasing frequency: lichen scrophulosorum. This is an allergy which mainly afflicts teenagers. Colonies of tiny nodes form on the skin, covered with yellowish-brownish flakes. Many a time this disease is wrongly diagnosed as acne.

Another very unpleasant variety of cutaneous tuberculosis is lupus erythematodes. It forms reddish and yellowish blotches with a distinct rim. Flaking sets in; the course is chronic.

For all these varieties of the disease there is a therapy with constant, successful cures: application of an aloe emulsion. The emulsion is applied to the afflicted areas three times a day. If this treatment should not bring the desired result after 15 days, a complementary treatment should be applied as follows: every morning one injection of 1 ml of aloe extract subcutaneously. After an interval of 15 injection-free days, another phase of 12 days follows with one injection of 1 ml daily.

Even if the injection cure has been successful it should be repeated after one year in the same way in order to strengthen the body's defenses. Children from five years of age on receive the same treatment, but with injections of 0,5 ml instead of 1 ml.

Small children are often afflicted with primary cutaneous tuberculosis. With the doctor's permission they receive the same injection treatment with ampullas of 0,2 ml each, as otherwise aloe should not be injected prior to the fifth year.

During the disease an ample supply of oxygen is essential. Sunbaths can be especially recommended. The therapy must be complemented by a diet low in salt and plenty of raw fruit and vegetables.

Moreover, plenty of vitamin D should be given, also cod-liver oil, yeast, dates, mushrooms and tomatoes. Tomatoes are especially suitable because they also contain vitamins K and A. As it is difficult for the consumer to judge the quality of fresh tomatoes, the author advises tomato juice instead, which is available in pharmacies, drug stores and health-food stores. These juices are guaranteed to be biological-dynamical. The therapy is mainly influenced by yeast, which eliminates disturbances of cellular respiration and checks inflammations.

DISORDER OF CARDIAC RHYTHM

In the chapter on arteriosclerosis and other age-related diseases we reported about the beneficent influence of an injection therapy with aloe extract on the heart circulation system of elderly people. These therapy results are also valid for patients of other age groups. With all aloe treatments a beneficent influence on the heart rhythm has been noted, which in all cases observed has become normal. Clinical observations have demonstrated that aloe extract not only influences the activity of the enzymes in general, but invigorates the activity of the enzyme systems in the heart tissue in particular. Tissue respiration increases!

A number of diseases appear in the form of an inflammation or degeneration of the heart muscle. According to clinical reports, the influence of aloe injections on the function of the heart muscle is seen as very favorable: it initiates a stabilizing effect on the strength of the heart.

Clinical tests have shown that one or two cures with aloe-extract injections increased the electrical activity of the heart. The chapter on kidney diseases describes the positive influence of bio-stimulated aloe extract on kidney function. Kidney function is known to be in close correlation with the activity of heart and blood vessels. Therefore the decision of physicians concerning the therapy of patients with heart and circulation problems with aloe extract should be based on the realization that because of its broad spectrum this therapy can influence virtually all systems of the organism.

The dosage in the case of heart and circulation disorders must be prescribed on an individual basis by taking into account the universal history and condition of the patient. The basic principles are to be found among the therapy instructions at the end of the chapter »Arteriosclerosis and Other Age-Related Diseases«.

It has been generally accepted that the aloe-injection cures bring about a noticeable lowering of a high cholesterol level in the blood. One patient from Berlin, born in 1911, experienced a complete normalization of her cholesterol level after the third cure with aloe extract, even though before the treatment it had been much too high. It must be noted that the patient in no way altered her life style and did not cut down on butter and other fats. Needless to say, such a positive influence on the lowering of the cholesterol level by the aloe therapy is more durable if the patient follows a diet. In the case of the above-mentioned patient, who is to be counted among the older generation, the blood-sugar value was also normalized. This can be traced back to the invigorating influence of the biogenic stimulators on the function of the pancreas.

In this connection we would like to recommend that changes of the blood-sugar values in the blood count be noted after an aloe therapy. In case of positive changes the physician would thus have a natural means of using the therapy in the case of diabetes mellitus.

MENINGITIS

As yet the precise causes of the illness of the spider-web skin, which, together with the layer of skin containing the cerebral vessels, forms the cerebral membrane, have not been determined. The scientific term for this disease is arachnoiditis, a dangerous variety of meningitis, which is often the consequence of nasopharyngitis.

Indications are a blistery rash at the mouth, heightened reflexes, eye tremulations with pupils of different sizes, vomiting along with acute dizziness, unbearable headache, fits of shivering with pains in all the muscles. Meningitis is infectious and dangerous to life. Even when cured completely a disposition to headaches, even deafness, tends to remain, and frequently paralysis. The doctor invariably prescribes antibiotics. In cases where life is endangered this is indispensable. In less serious cases, however, and after danger to life is past, the aloe-extract cure should be used, because it stabilizes the healing process and reinvigorates the weakened immune system.

The following therapy instructions apply:

For thirty days one daily injection of 1 ml each to be applied subcutaneously (forearm) in the morning hours, to be followed by a period of rest. After an interval of 30 days without injections, the cure is completed with 30 more injections, i.e. 1 ml once a day.

IMPOTENCY (POTENCY OF THE MAN)

Potency problems appear with increasing frequency; they are functional disturbances of the man which, it is interesting to note, do not make themselves felt just in the so-called best years, but already afflict very young men. It is this phenomenon which points to psychic correlations. Man is basically sensitive; through constant exposure to stimuli and stress situations, his mind is so strained that certain subtle stimulants are received in an imperfect or distorted way. The psychologists are to a great extent consulted by men from 30 on up with problems of potency. This is not the place to deal with individual problems of partnership, which belong in the office of a psychologist. We just want to state some general principles how the inadequate or interrupted potency can be made to function normally again. It goes without saying that the patient's expectation of fulfillment can only be realized if he is able to attain a close partnership before receiving organic aid.

As we know, the term impotency comprises not only the failure of the man to reach and retain the erection of the penis, which is necessary for completing sexual intercourse, but also sterility, i.e. his complete inability of procreation. The therapy recommended below can only be of help for restoring the ability of erection. Readers of the fundamental articles of this publication will not be surprised to find an aloe cure recommended here. The introductory statements have made clear that the working mechanism of an aloe therapy functions via the central nervous system. It has been emphasized that the course of life, the whole motivation of the patient, the invigoration of his interest and his activities are positively influenced by the biogenic stimulators, even at an advanced age. In 1972 the Russian physician Dr. Batrak for the first time employed the tissue therapy according to Prof. Filatow. He was to treat patients in the beginning stages of impaired cerebral circulation, of neurasthenia, of vegetative dystonia, which in all patients were accompanied by pronounced sexual deficiency.

The patients were men between 55 and 72. In all cases the therapy proved effective by improving the general condition, restoring sleep, and increasing intellectual and physical ability — that is to say, the ability to work; restlessness, irritability and the feeling of weakness decreased. Some men experienced an improvement of their sexual potency, others found this potency restored.

Similar successes have been reported by Dr. Weinstein, who has been using the method of Prof. Filatow since 1961.

Our present state of knowledge makes the following aloe cure advisable:

Twice a week, preferably in the middle and at the end, 1 ml each of bio-stimulated aloe extract is to be injected subcutaneously, i.e. under the skin of the thigh. The cure should last for three months, comprising altogether 24 — 26 injections. During this time one teaspoon of Damiana Urtinktur should be taken undiluted every morning after breakfast. After the cure Damiana can be taken for two more months unless it produces an undesired effect of excessive libido. If necessary the cure can be repeated once a year.

Damiana Urtinktur is available without prescription in the pharmacy.

SCIATICA

This very painful affliction, also called neuritis ischiadica, is a neuralgia of the nervus ischiadicus. Formerly the following causes were seen as being primarily responsible: consequences of infections (influenza, decayed teeth, tonsilitis), colds and spinal changes. Lately, metabolic disturbances, among them rheumatism, have been diagnosed as causes with increasing frequency. Quite often, lack of vitamin B is responsible. In many cases, endogenic poisons can trigger the disease, such as diabetes mellitus with its latent varieties; increased blood sugar alone can trigger the disease. Not only endogenic poisons, i.e. those produced by the body itself, can be responsible, but also exogenic poisons: breathing in toxic substances, as well as excessive use of tobacco and alcohol. The aloe therapy is successful with all varieties of sciatica which have not been caused by infections. The prospects are especially high when the disease has been caused by changes in the spinal column and by the above-mentioned poisons.

The following therapy with bio-stimulated aloe extract is recommended:

Every other day one injection of 1 ml each subcutaneously into the thigh for patients up to the age of about 60; the first cure phase comprises 30 injections; after an injection-free period of 30 days the second cure phase follows with altogether 15 injections (every other day 1 ml). With patients over 60 the first cure phase comprises 15 injections; after an injection-free interval of 30 days, 15 more injections follow. Here again the injections of 1 ml each are administered every other day.

CANCER OF THE THROAT

In this case, the aloe cure has effected at least the stagnation of the disease! Compared to the helplessness of previous therapies this is quite an achievement!

Cancer of the throat can be caused by excessive smoking of cigarettes. In many cases we find a different variety of this cancer, which infects the larynx from the esophagus, from the throat or from the rim of the tongue. Symptoms are permanent hoarseness and tiring quickly in conversation. Academic medicine knows only laryngotracheotomy.

It is indispensable if the doctor can see no other way. But patients are well advised to consult two different doctors independently. Prior to a laryngotracheotomy, a responsible physician will try biological remedies to effect a cure without such a radical operation.

We advise doctors to try the therapies listed in the following chapter.

LARYNGOPHTHISIS (TUBERCULOSIS OF THE LARYNX)

This disease has become comparatively rare. Its most famous victim was the German Emperor Friedrich III, who in 1888, the so-called »year of three emperors«, ruled for only 90 days and with his peace plans opposed Bismarck's power politics; Bismarck wanted to dethrone the irksome Hohenzollern regent on account of »incurable illness«. The monarch communicated with the people around him by means of written notes. At the time, the Emperor's disease was in fact incurable, and it brought about his death.

The most frequent cause is tuberculosis of the lungs . . .

The first symptoms are a husky voice, hoarseness, to be followed by difficulties in swallowing, the urge to cough, and shortness of breath. An examination always diagnoses swelling of the larynx and large nodes on one half of the larynx.

The therapy consists of:

---

1. Solar radiation of the larynx
2. Compresses with warm olive oil around the throat
3. Injections with aloe extract as follows:
   Subcutaneous injections into the thigh in the morning hours of 30 consecutive days, to be followed by 15 – 20 minutes of rest. After an injection-free interval of 30 days, 30 more injections are given, 1 ml a day.
   After one year the cure is to be repeated.

BONE FRACTURES, INJURIES AND ABSCESSES

In case of open, festering bone fractures, burns of all kinds, inflamed trophic wounds (trophic = caused by nutritional disturbances), in case of infected injuries, abscesses from various causes, as well as cuts of all kinds, the application of aloe juice (succus aloes) helps. The contents are as follows: out of 100 ml, 80 ml are a watery solution from bio-stimulated juice pressed from freshly harvested aloe leaves; the other 20 ml are ethanol, 95 % proof.

In this case biological medicine can prove popular medicine right. In grandmother's family-medicine chest and, even more simply, on grandmother's flower board, there was aloe, the »first-aid plant«. If someone cut himself while shaving or peeling potatoes, the viscous juice was pressed from an aloe leaf and immediately applied to the wound. Whoever doubts this should try it out himself. The plant does provide highly effective first aid. The wound closes immediately and heals quickly. The plant even cures itself: when the leaf is broken off the stem (lower leaves are best!), the scar on the stem closes and the juice stops flowing. Popular medicine ascribed all this to a constringent effect.

But now we know that it is more than this astringency. The healing power is derived from the biogenic stimulators, a complete, self-contained enzyme system.

With the above-mentioned indications the following therapy is recommended:

One or two teaspoons of bio-stimulated aloe juice are applied to the injured areas until they are healed. With injuries and cuts one treatment will frequently suffice. In more complicated cases a therapy of two or three weeks is adequate. The first healing effects, however, appear very early.

CANCER

Only a biological therapy can be universally successful defense against cancer. Even though academic medicine now concedes that biological treatment should accompany conventional forms of medicine such as chemotherapy, ray treatment and surgery, the change of attitude toward biological therapy must be more fundamental. Biological defense against cancer must take first place, in other words the opposite of what has been hitherto postulated. It is the conventional methods, which, if necessary, must complement biological cancer therapy. This is not a mere quarrel about priorities, but an insight into the phenomenon of man's illness in his universality. For decades, the cancer researcher Dr. Josef Issels has been of this conviction and states that first of all the body's defenses, i.e. man's immune system, must be mobilized against cancer. Admittedly, many cancer patients do not respond to radiology and hospital medicine any more, mainly those at painfully advanced stages. They can be helped only by immune therapy. By and large, conservative cancer therapies can be no more than cancer treatment, whereas the object should be not only to eliminate the tumor, but also its cause. We should not forget that in traditional medicine not only cancer cells are affected, but also healthy cells can be destroyed.

Cancer cells are not diseased body cells, but cells of the cancer, i.e. new cells multiplying. The cancerous growth is a self-contained entity which independently forms new cells. These anti-cells crowd in on the healthy body cells, and that is the actual instigation of the cancerous process. It must be said that by no means should we revert to the other extreme, i.e. seeing the cancer in psychic terms only. If, for instance, a patient's disposition or habitually wrong nutrition have brought about a disease of his stomach, where food often remains for hours and thus exerts unusually strong pressure on the gastric membranes and walls, in the long run this can lead to cancer, unless the body's defenses are able to cope with this situation.

For the biological cancer therapy healthful nutrition is of utmost importance. But what is healthful nutrition? First of all: reasonable nutrition! That means eating moderately, but regularly. Meat and sausage should be rare items on the menu. Sugar, jams, smoked food as well as salt-cured meat should not be consumed at all. Instead the menu should consist mainly of vegetarian food rich in bulkage, above all whole-grain products, fresh vegetables, salads, fruit. Healthful nutrition activates the metabolism. This has a beneficent effect on the body's defenses. According to Prof. Leitzmann from the Justus-Liebig University in Giessen, 45 % of all cancer cases are caused by deficient nutrition. In this context we would like to recommend freshly pressed juices as an important nutritional complement, most emphatically the so-called red juices from red beets, cherries, blueberries, black currants, elderberries and blackberries. Also yellow beets, which contain carotin (same as carrots), celery (containing phosphorus) and radishes are important.

In short: the body's own cells can live on these juices; the cancer cells cannot. Why are the red juices so essential?

The lack of red dye is inducive to cancer. With an adequate supply of red dye the respiration of the body's cells is enhanced and their resistance is increased. As we can see from this example, old lore is proved right again.

The red vegetable dyes are of utmost importance for detoxicating the organism, because oxidation processes destroy toxins. Furthermore, the red plant dyes positively influence cellular respiration and capillary permeability. If these juices are taken regularly the red plant dyes exert a curative effect, strengthened by important attendant substances, among them minerals, vitamins and enzymes. Dr. Seeger, eminent cancer researcher in the G.D.R., has been using the juice of red beets in his biological cancer therapy for decades; so has R. A. Hoffmann, the well known practitioner of biological medicine.

He noted that one litre (i.e. appr. a quart) of pressed juice provides the patient with 1000 gamma of oxygen.

Therefore the cancer patient is well advised to drink three quarters of a litre of juice pressed from red beets (health-food store) daily. He should always remember that lack of oxygen is inducive to cancer.

Both Hoffmann and Dr. Seeger and the author of this publication have noted during various therapies that the effect of preserved juices is therapeutically negligible. Therefore: **Use only freshly pressed juices!** Fresh fruit biologically grown is available in almost all health-food stores. The most advantageous method is pressing the juice with the usual household appliances and drinking them fresh!

CANCER AND THE PSYCHE

From old Tibetan medicine it is known that the autopsies of old men showed them to have had testicular cancer without the decisive process of cell division having taken place. In these cases the immune system had been strong enough to arrest cell division. With cancer, the system of the body's defenses is one of the key questions. Wherever serious diseases, constant apprehension, psychic stress situations such as mourning, sorrow, or existential anxieties have weakened the immune system or even caused its breakdown, the cancer cells can begin their excrescent growth. Therefore all therapies ought to pay heed to the psychic and physical components of the patient as well as his inborn immune system.

Even short, but intense stress situations can cause the immune system to fail completely. Infections and other diseases can cause the conditions which in most cases can lead to a catastrophy. It has been noted that people who had been through very difficult times and mental crises were afflicted by several diseases at the same time, such as cancer, diabetes insipidus, meningitis, to name just a few, because their immune system had been weakened. The American Space Agency has made an interesting statement concerning the function of the immune system. According to the newspaper »Welt am Sonntag« of December 2, 1984, the instruments in the control center of Cape Canaveral registered that during the critical phase of re-entry into the atmosphere of the earth the immune system of the astronauts was temporarily paralyzed. This shows that even very short periods of tension prior to decisive experiences and other abnormal cases of stress can paralyze the whole immune system. This makes clear how much worse the effect of continuous stress must be on it. As a consequence, the body's defenses usually break down. And these are the conditions that favor the development of cancer. It is a similar precondition as for AIDS.

Prof. Bialock from the University of Galveston, Texas, has proved the correlation between man's mental state and his immune system: he explains the interdependence between psyche and immune system with a hormonal chain reaction. According to this thesis the cerebral cortex transmits the stress impulse in case of anxieties and similar tensions to the hypothalamus (part of the mid-brain). »From there, chemical messengers are dispatched to the pituary gland, which then produces a fountain of hormones«, as Prof. Bialock has found.

The renewal of the production of hormones enables the body to make up for the deficits of the immune system; this restores the body's ability to wage the defensive war against the excrescent growth of the cancer cells. If during heavy stress a hormonal chain reaction sets in, the biogenic stimulators from the aloe act as a counterforce to restore the hormonal depot. Moreover, the injections of bio-stimulated aloe extract strengthen the vital defenses, so that the cancer patient's resistance against other diseases is increased. It is the peculiar influence of the aloe that the effect of specific anti-cancer drugs is increased.

Cancer cells disintegrating under the influence of anti-cancer drugs can form toxins. This poses the danger of poisoning. Injected aloe extract has an anti-toxic effect. Therefore aloe-injection cures can be recommended along with anti-cancer compounds.

In light of these facts the aloe therapy complements cancer treatment. The dosage must be fixed by the doctor. The following therapy is recommended:

In the early stages of cancer:

For 30 consecutive days one daily injection of 1 ml of aloe extract subcutaneously (thigh); after an interval of 30 days, 30 more injections follow: once a day one ampulla of 1 ml.

At an advanced stage:

For 12 consecutive days one daily ampulla of 1 ml each to be injected under the skin; after an injection-free interval of 15 days, one daily ampulla of 0,5 ml to be injected for 12 consecutive days. After a pause of 30 days one daily ampulla of 1 ml to be injected for four consecutive days.

In the two following years the cure should be repeated as above.

When applying the aloe therapy in the treatment of cancer it is essential to note that in this system the battle of the body's defenses is based on the organization of the antibodies. Dr. Sadychow reports that with 13 out of 27 patients who had received 20 — 30 injections with bio-stimulated aloe extract for the general stimulation of their defenses, so-called irregular antibodies developed in the blood. That means: antibodies without any regularity, i.e. irregular antibodies, are immune antibodies. During the above-mentioned clinical research they showed up in **all blood groups**. These findings demonstrate that biological therapies can be an important complementation of conservative cancer medicine.

LEISHMANIA

This disease has its name from the English military doctor Sir William Leishman (1885 — 1926). Several variations are known. Whereas in former times the different forms of leishmania were mainly Oriental diseases and were not especially dreaded in Europe, with the exception of Russia and the Balkans, they have lately become more wide-spread as a consequence of mass tourism to far-away lands. The disease can be triggered by the sting of a certain species of mosquito, but also by infections through contaminated food or through contact with stray dogs, which are carriers of certain insects. This disease not only causes node-shaped rashes and furuncular growths, but also damages spleen, liver and bone marrow.

This affliction ought to be taken seriously and immediately checked by an aloe-injection cure. Treatment as follows:

On 30 consecutive days one daily ampulla of 1 ml each to be injected subcutaneously (thigh); after a 30-day period of rest, the second cure phase with 30 daily injections (1 ml each) follows.

Moreover, aloe emulsion should be rubbed lightly into the afflicted areas, twice a day for two weeks.

LEPROSY

Leprosy is one of the most dreadful scourges to afflict mankind from prehistoric times well into the days of high civilization.

According to current estimates, between 8 and 10 million people are afflicted at present and live in dire misery.

Leprosy is a chronic, infectious disease with an incubation time of between two and thirty years. Rods comparable to the bacilli of tuberculosis infest the human body in great numbers. The causative organism is called mycobacterium leprae; it was discovered in 1873 by the Norwegian physician Dr. C. A. Hansen (1841 – 1912). After him the leprosy colonies in many places were called »Hansen stations«.

In general leprosy appears in two variations: a nervous leprosy which causes a severe weakening of the whole organism; and as node or skin leprosy, which results in open wounds and an increasing decomposition of the living body. The first symptoms are red blotches on the skin, which develop into festering ulcers, break open, and gradually distort the facial expression of its victim in a horrible way. At an advanced stage the limbs begin to waste away and atrophy: the fingers become paralyzed and fall off, so that of the hands only stumps remain; with the feet it is similar. The terrible disease attacks all organs. Among others the palate becomes distorted, later it disappears completely, which makes eating difficult. The destruction of nasal bones and cartilage lead to complete ruin of the face. Frequently ulcers in the eye-balls break open and cause the eyes to run out.

The lepers degenerate into helpless creatures; frequently they are brutally abandoned by their fellows – even in our time! – because the smell of their disease and the sight of their tortures become unbearable.

In 13th-century Europe there were still 20.000 institutions sheltering leprosy patients. By the 18th century leprosy had been conquered in Europe, thanks to universal hygienic measures.

Even in ancient Europe the fate of lepers used to be ghastly. They lived outside human society, outside the protection of the law. These people in their dire misery were not allowed to leave the leprosy hospital. They had to warn healthy people approaching them by means of a hand rattle, a gruesome signal of creeping death. Overseas, lepers were simply left to their primitive fate.

In the past 100 years much has been done for leprosy patients throughout the world, especially in social respects. Major contributions have been made by leprosy organizations, missions of churches, and health organizations, above all the WHO. But still there are heart-rending instances of contacts with newly abandoned patients. Here is an example: Sister Maria Regina from the Sichili Hospital, P.O. Mulobezi, Via Livingstone, Zambia (formerly Southern Rhodesia), Africa, writes in a letter to the author of this publication:

»At the moment so many poor people come to our station, because there is hunger everywhere. This is a vital threat to the lepers who no longer have hands or feet, because they cannot earn a living. I am grateful for any little gift. Lately we had a few very serious cases of leprosy, and last week an old man asked to be accepted. He had neither hands nor feet left. In his young years he had been a chief – but when he got leprosy he became an outcast; when he developed open wounds and one limb after the other fell off he was simply abandoned. They took him into the bush, and there he would have starved had it not been for a man from the saw-mill who happened to pass by looking for trees. Today he has recuperated enough that he can at least eat everything again. Much more ought to be done for these miserable people here, but we alone cannot do it.«

The brave Catholic nun is only too right. These eight to ten million leprosy patients all over the world need international solidarity and active help. We should not simple care for them in their misery, but cure them. This is a general commandment formulated as a law concerning leprosy as early as in the Old Testament (Moses, 3/14).

Again we are dealing with a disease with its roots in the social misery, in the breakdown of the immune system. These suffering people ought to receive lasting help through the aloe healing system, wherever it is not yet too late.

In face of the fact that the aloe, the medicinal plant with its curative compounds, originates in the home country of these same lepers and thrives there in ideal, so-called medicinal quality, without man knowing about this natural resource, we cannot help being shocked at the simple fact that civilization is about to exploit the earth, but has not been able to realize one of the first commandments of creation: »Make yourselves masters over the earth.«

Here, more so than with other diseases, the aloe-extract therapy must take into account the generally weakened constitution of the leprosy patient.

Therefore we recommend as a general rule:

At first every other day one injection of 0,5 ml of aloe extract subcutaneously (thigh); altogether 30 injections. After an injection-free interval of 30 days a second cure phase follows with a daily dose of 0,5 ml, administered as above. If this first cure proves successful it should be continued after one year with a daily ampulla of 1 ml to be injected on 30 consecutive days.

The usual interval of 30 days without injections follows. Then 30 more daily injections of 1 ml each.

If the first cure phase has not arrested the disease, it is to be repeated: every other day 0,5 ml; altogether, including the interval, the second cure lasts for 150 days. In this case the second cure series should bring about an amelioration of the general condition, so that in the third year the basic cure can be administered.

Besides, the patient should be treated with aloe emulsion; at the beginning, aloe emulsion should be rubbed lightly into the afflicted areas, twice a day over a period of 30 days. The treatment with emulsion is to be repeated every other month.

This emulsion ought to be stocked in every doctor's office and mission station of developing countries, as it is not only an effective, but also cheap medicament, which should help to resocialize these seriously ill people and thus save expenses in countries which must operate with the greatest economy. The possible scope of this new therapy is demonstrated by the number of patients, i.e. 8 − 10 million throughout the world, who are outside the work force and need costly care.

MULTIPLE SCLEROSIS

According to accepted belief this ailment belongs to the diseases of the nervous system, which is correct. Spinal marrow and brain are affected. But it is often overlooked that through an apparent programming defect within the central nervous system a dysregulation of the vasomotorium is a concomitant indication. It is this dysregulation in the sense of the Winiwarter-Bürger disease, with inflamed cellular conglomerations and tissue densification along the artery walls leading to a restriction in the flow of blood, which also has to be counteracted in the case of multiple sclerosis. Therefore the prime object of any treatment must be to increase blood circulation. For the simple reason that the Winiwarter-Bürger disease is an inflammation, it can be a precursor of multiple sclerosis. The author of this publication considers it important that the correlation be thoroughly researched, because this can lead to the discovery of what causes multiple sclerosis as a first step toward finding a cure.

The symptoms of multiple sclerosis are spastic forms of paralysis in the legs, difficulties in walking, trembling hands, tremulation of the eyeballs, breakdown of reflexes, urethral and intestinal obstruction as well as heavy depressions alternating in a striking manner with compulsive fits of weeping and laughing. Between these spells even patients of multiple sclerosis may experience periods of a sanguine and cheerful mood. It is exactly these »sunny, cheerful days« that are characteristic of multiple sclerosis and most persuasively point up the serious correlation with the central nervous system. In some respects the patient behaves like a hysteric.

According to academic medicine the causes of multiple sclerosis are unknown; therefore the author would like to state some facts which point to a psychosomatic background: with a majority of patients of multiple sclerosis, serious and persistent tensions in their partnerships, negative − including traumatic − experiences in their sexual lives were noted; these led to depressive moods and increasing isolation, moreover to social protest against their immediate surroundings, often in connection with an unresolved Oedipus complex. As a result of his social protest against disappointing experiences, deprivation of love and tenderness, the patient begins to isolate himself more and more in his disease. Admittedly this thesis sounds shocking; nevertheless the author recommends that the patients of multiple sclerosis be analyzed through hypnosis, and he is convinced that in many cases this thesis will prove true. People who are susceptible to this disease, especially those with difficulties of adaptation, with problems when leaving the home of their parents, are characterized by an originally subconscious, later on conscious, manifest attitude of denial; in the central nervous system this effects such a reprogramming, such radical changes that the ailment is triggered. Whereas patients of a different disposition fall victim to a breakdown of the immune system and eventually to cancer if confronted with grave psychic changes caused by disappointments and worries, by anxieties and persistent excitement, another type of patient tends more to nervous diseases with a possibility of multiple sclerosis. It is remarkable that this disease frequently afflicts young people with psychic problems such as the ones described above.

Aloe extract plays a decisive part in re-aligning the central nervous system, stimulating the defenses and vitality in general.

Aloe injection cures with patients of multiple sclerosis have for a number of years arrested, in some cases even improved or cured, the disease, if it had been correctly diagnosed in time. For this reason we would like to recommend a therapy which should give many patients of multiple sclerosis hope, bring about improvement, and perhaps even change their lives considerably.

For 30 consecutive days 1 ml of aloe extract is to be injected daily under the skin of the thigh. After an injection-free interval of 30 days the second cure phase follows with 30 more injections to be administered daily, preferably in the morning hours.

If this does not effect a noticeable improvement of the general condition, the cure should be repeated after one year, and again in yearly intervals, altogether four repetitions.

Concomitant measures are very important. A change of diet is imperative.

Based on our experience we recommend a special diet that we have chosen from many possibilities. It is the diet according to Prof. Dr. Brauchle:

»Keep a strict raw vegetarian diet over a period of months, in addition to wheat sprouts or freshly germinated grain, especially in times of sudden deterioration of the disease« (health-food store). For the duration of the aloe cure, i.e. 90 days, we recommend this raw vegetarian diet in connection with a number of fresh juices rich in vitamins — with the exception of cauliflower and rhubarb.

Alcohol, coffee, black tea, mustard, salt, sugar, vinegar and pepper are strictly forbidden.

East Indian kidney tea is to be recommended.

Partial sunbaths, relaxing massages and gymnastics are important, so that gait, mobility and grasping motions can be improved. The patient must be treated with great care; strain of all kinds is to be avoided. Otherwise serious relapses ensue.

This treatment should be accompanied by a psychological influence on the patient: he must be encouraged, his confidence in his organism and vitality must be carefully built up. He should be made to realize that there is a prospect of arresting his ailment, even a cure. Furthermore it is important that the psychologist and the attending doctor direct their mental-psychological work toward helping the patient establish a functioning partnership.

After every aloe cure, treatment with Recarcin (pharmacy) in the form of capsules and ointment are recommended.

Dr. Meljankow and Dr. Rjabinina, the Russian doctors from Minsk who for a long time had been working according to the method of Prof. Filatow, reported as early as 1958 about successful cures in the case of multiple sclerosis. The title of their report: »The Use of Tissue Therapy with Diseases of the Nervous System.«

Moreover, a stay at a sanatorium in an area above 2000 feet rich in forests is to be recommended once a year.

NEURITIS

One variation of neuritis is rather wide-spread: polyneuritis. This is a general inflammation of numerous nerves, which triggers disturbances of the paths of motorial or sensory conduction of the nervous system, sometimes of both. There also exists a degenerative form of this disease. Polyneuritis is often mistaken for multiple sclerosis. In the same way as with that disease, the muscles degenerate at an advanced stage, sinew reflexes decrease and eventually disappear. Typical symptoms are impaired gait, paralysis in legs and arms, palpitation of the heart, profuse perspiration, nerve cords and muscles cause a great deal of pain.

The following therapy is to be used:

> 1. Change of diet with special emphasis on raw vegetarian food, preferably fruit and vegetables with a high vitamin B content (carrots, tomatoes etc.)
> 2. Air baths; with inflammations decreasing also sun baths
> 3. Massages, first of non-afflicted areas, later also of inflamed ones.
> 4. Packs and medical baths
> 5. Injections cure with aloe extract as follows:
>
>   Every other day one ampulla of 1 ml each to be injected under the skin (thigh) in the early morning hours, to be followed by 15 minutes of rest before breakfast; the first cure phase consists of altogether 15 injections. No injections for the following 20 days. After this, 15 more injections of 1 ml each to be administered every other day.
>
>   After nine months the cure should be repeated.

Polyneuritis can be caused by excessive use of alcohol, nicotine and chemical drugs. Sometime the disease is a consequence of diphtheria. Other causes can be poisoning through carbon oxide as well as arsenic. Moreover, lead and sulfohydrogen toxication can trigger nerve inflammations of this kind. Also diabetes, smallpox, malaria and even influenza can cause neuritis.

With its special anti-toxic effect, an aloe-extract cure will bring about constant, successful results.

NEURODERMITIS

This comprises several forms of eczema which originate in the body itself (i.e. endogenic), or may develop from the disposition of the body, but not through external influences. According to the research of Dr. Vaitl, patients with obvious allergy factors as well as problems of nutrition and metabolism had the following psycho-syndrome: »increased irritability, a tendency toward isolation with depressive, disgruntled moods, a strong bond to the mother, and masochist tendencies. These psychic causes have a decisive influence on the recurrence as well as the disappearance of the disease, without being necessarily themselves the triggering psychic cause of the disease.« This conforms exactly with the author's findings. With this type of patient it is always the metabolism based on deficient nutrition which triggers the disease. The patient is a nervous eater; in a depressive mood he gulps down his food; eating is almost a compensation for sexual discontent. The basic therapy must be of a psychological nature. The patient must have the chance to talk his problems over. This conversation therapy must be concentrated exclusively on the patient. It should be like a talk among equals rather than a questioning session. The patient should not see himself in the role of an afflicted person, but of a client making friends with a more experienced person.

This conversation therapy is accompanied by a course of treatment with aloe extract with its stimulation of the central nervous system.

The following therapy is recommended:

> 30 injections of aloe extract, 1 ml each, to be administered subcutaneously (thigh) every other day. After an interval of 30 days the second cure phase of 30 injections follows, every other day one injection as above.

During the disease aloe emulsion can be applied as a complement. Nutrition rich in raw vegetarian food is recommended. After completion of the cure, stinging-nettle juice should be drunk three times a day for a period of six months. If the inflammations ooze, dry healing earth (pharmacy) should be applied instead of aloe emulsion.

KIDNEY DISEASES

Clinical and experimental analyses of the recent past prove the curative influence of aloe compounds on kidney function, which is essential for the functioning of heart and vessels. Medical reports have been published which attest to the dynamic changes of the functional condition of the kidneys, even with older people, as a result of the aloe therapy. According to these reports, the therapy stimulates the kidneys appreciably; this stimulation concerns both the intrarenal blood circulation (i.e. circulation in the kidneys themselves) and the excreting function of the kidneys. The reports state furthermore that the therapy activates the flow of blood through the kidneys and increases the speed of glomerulo-filtration, i.e. natural dialysis, or »rinsing of the kidneys«; after three aloe cures the patients undergoing the treatment experienced an increase in glomerulo-filtration of 150 %. Not only was the intrarenal blood circulation improved but also the excretion of nitrogen. In an experiment to examine the effect of the therapy on patients of two different age groups — the one between 50 and 59, the other between 60 and 74 — the attending doctors noted that with the older group the therapy effected stronger stimulation than with the younger one. Positive changes of kidney function are a consequence of improved metabolism within the kidneys. The essential part of the aloe therapy is the beneficent influence of its active agents on the renicapsular tissue.

When we consider that for seriously ill kidney patients the prospects of a cure through academic medicine as well as natural remedies have been rather dim, the introduction of the aloe therapy into medical practice can be justifiably called a positive breakthrough. A system as complicated as the kidneys is susceptible to many kinds of stress and manifold diseases. In his therapy the attending doctor must differentiate carefully. Therefore we recommend the basic therapy as follows:

Twice a week 1 ml of bio-stimulated aloe extract is injected subcutaneously into the thigh, until 30 injections have been reached. After an injection-free interval of 30 days, the second cure phase (same as the first one) follows. After another interval of 30 days and the final cure phase, altogether 90 ampullas will have been injected.

The injection should be administered in the morning hours.

This basic rule applies only to adults. The kidney diet must be strictly salt-free. A raw vegetarian diet is always advisable. If the cure proves successful, protein-foods can be added to the diet. The therapy can be effectively complemented by a tea mixture of bean pods, ortosiphon and rose hips.

Furthermore the therapy can be enhanced by horse-radish distillates, because horse radish increases blood circulation in the kidneys.

OZENA

Quite a sonorous name for a malodorous disease of the nose! The term »stink nose« is generally better known. It is fully justified. A really evil stench emanates from the afflicted nose. It is a consequence of the bacterial breakdown of the scabs, which form in the nose on account of inflammations. The following treatment is advisable:

Aloe-injection cure: 15 injections to be administered subcutaneously (under the skin), 1 ml daily. After an interval of 12 days, 15 more injections.

PSORIASIS

Psoriasis is caused by very unspecific changes. Among typical causes we find neurotic tendencies, especially existential anxiety, fear of punishment, the so-called »bad conscience«, and above all inferiority complexes. Psoriasis often leads to loss of hair and complete baldness. Its course is long drawn out and marked by relapses. Sometimes it is caused by metabolic disturbances. It can also develop in connection with diabetes, in which case the itching becomes unbearable.

The best that can be effected by ointments and ray therapy of conventional medicine is a superficial healing and a temporary disappearance of the scales. But this is not a real cure, because the actual causes have not been eliminated; they are to be found in a disturbed information apparatus of the central nervous system. This is where treatment should begin.

The following therapy is recommended:

1. Injection cure: 1 ml of aloe extract to be injected daily on 30 consecutive days subcutaneously (thigh) in the morning hours. After an interval of 30 days, the second part of the cure follows, 30 days, same as above. The cure can be repeated after one year.
2. Absolutely no nicotine and alcohol during the disease. Table salt is to be substituted by sea salt; oil and fats to be used sparingly (no butter; instead: sunflower margarine).
3. During treatment the diet should mainly consist of raw vegetarian food, especially green salads, horse radishes and red radishes.
4. Sunbaths

PSYCHICAL DISEASES OF THE SKIN

ACNE

In many cases the different forms of acne vulgaris torment the mostly juvenile patients so persistently, because the psychosomatic background is not analyzed.

As the outer-most layer of the human individual, the skin is the predestined organ for expressing emotional phenomena. Blushing and getting pale belong here as well as the so-called goose bumps. As we can see, a whole number of psychic processes are responsible for disturbing the functional mechanism between glands of the skin and vessels. Acne is a disturbance of the secretion of the sebaceous glands. It appears from the beginning of puberty to about the 25th year of life. If adults above this age are still afflicted by acne, it is usually caused by retarded maturing both sexually and emotionally, i.e. concerning the harmony of moods and drives such as pleasure, displeasure, anger, happiness or sadness. These emotions are not balanced, not resolved. As a consequence, mental conflicts develop. Non-realized drives can often trigger acne by disturbing the function of the sebaceous glands. Acne can also be caused by deficient nutrition, such as excessive amounts of pork, eggs, bacon etc. Metabolic byproducts are no longer eliminated through the skin as necessary.

There is another, especially unpleasant form of acne which afflicts female patients. After squeezing or scratching damages the skin, lentil-size flat scars develop, which become easily inflamed. These cases can be seen as auto-aggressions, self-punishment, protest against the immediate surroundings (parents, teachers etc.). These aggressions are coercive, and with neurotic patients serve to let off steam.

With acne the following therapy is recommended:

1. For 12 consecutive days aloe emulsion is to be applied to the afflicted areas once a day (before bedtime).
2. At the same time, aloe extract is to be injected: 15 injections of 1 ml each subcutaneously (thigh); the first four injections at daily intervals; from the fifth injection on one every other day in the morning hours. An injection-free interval of 20 days follows. The second cure phase also comprises 15 injections, to be given at daily intervals.
3. During the interval and after the cure, stinging-nettle juice from the health-food store, drug store or pharmacy should be taken three times a day (morning, noon, evening); mind the instructions on the package! This cure conforms to the course of ailment; it should be observed throughout puberty.

CHRONIC NETTLE RASH

Urticaria is caused by suppressed aggressions as well as masochist and exhibitionist inclinations. Neurotic tensions erupt in demonstrative protest against the immediate surroundings, mostly against withdrawal of love and lack of affection. The patient stimulates a kind of self-punishment. As the organ of contact and expression, the skin plays a dominant role.

The causes will have to be attacked by psychological treatment. Besides, we recommend a cure with aloe extract, which ought to be explained to the patient with special psychological care. He should be told that it works via the central nervous system and will initiate a normalization of the process of information emanating from there. Nettle rash can also be triggered by medicinal toxins as well as allergies against certain plants and animals. An allergy test is always advisable. Often it is an allergy against strawberries.

With psychic and organic causes — aloe extract is most successfully used in cases of intoxication — an injection cure is recommended:

---

15 aloe-extract injections of 1 ml each are administered subcutaneously (thigh); the first four at daily intervals, the rest every other day. After a pause of 20 days, the second cure phase with another 15 injections follows, one injection a day.

The diet should be low in salt with plenty of fruit and vegetables; no strawberries!

RHEUMATISM

The term rheumatism comprises various diseases of the connective tissue. It comes from ancient Greek and means »flowing«, which is quite descriptive of the symptoms: the pains do flow through the different organs of the body, they move around and appear in various forms as inflammation pains. If we want to understand these disagreeable pains moving through the whole body, we must visualize the structure of the connective tissue. It is an intricate mesh of fine perfection which is to be found in all organs and as a supportive structure gives the body its firmness and shape. Therefore, if the connective tissue becomes defective, the disease can penetrate into all parts of the body. Thus the many rheumatic ailments can develop, e.g. rheumatism of the muscles, of the joints or the spinal column, to name just a few. The classification of rheumatic diseases follows the diagnostic-therapeutic characteristics, and the air names were coined by the International League of Rheumatism in Toronto in 1957.

In face of the fact that rheumatism can be a life-long illness precluding the ability to work and leading to early sickliness, it becomes evident that society should make every therapeutic and hygienic effort in fighting a problem of this eminent social importance.

The most frequent forms of rheumatism are probably caused by bacteria entering the blood stream, e.g. chronic angina as well as defective or dead teeth. As there are no local complaints, no attention is paid; but these local suppurative focuses constantly let off bacterial poisons into the bloodstream, which are at first eliminated by the immune powers until one day the constantly overtaxed immune system becomes hyper-sensitive and the sometimes perennial stream of poisons throws the overburdened immune system off balance. As a reaction, a rheumatic inflammation breaks out. In many cases defective nutrition favours rheumatic diseases. Other causes can be the well-known catarrhal diseases, especially when neglected, as well as when the body temperature falls below normal, or chronically cold feet. In this context we would like to point out that chronically cold feet with their impaired circulation can be quickly and successfully treated with arnica ointment, which has an excellent deep-reaching effect.

In the author's opinion the fact that general exhaustion can also be the cause of a rheumatic disease is too little known. Constant stress and tension as well as the fear of not being able to solve the accumulating problems of daily life overtax the reactions of the central nervous system and reprogram it abnormally. Here we realize the correlation with the immune apparatus directed by the central nervous system, with the system of the body's defenses. Therefore any therapy ought to concentrate on normalizing the patient's life style, on eliminating factors conducive to disease! A purely medicinal treatment will not have enduring success unless the patient's life style has been positively influenced and his immune powers systematically rebuilt. Patients of rheumatism tend to be discouraged by previous prognoses, and therefore it is essential for the doctor to stress the psychological aspects of his therapy. In cases where the physician is overtaxed, this task can be taken over by the social community of the League of Rheumatism.

The question whether rheumatism is hereditary is often asked: a concern which to all practical purposes influences the patient's attitude toward his disease and his expectation concerning a cure from a psychic angle.

According to present-day knowledge, the disease itself is not hereditary. But on account of inherited weaknesses in certain respects there can be a disposition toward the disease, i.e. toward rheumatic reaction.

Now a combination of the compounds from bio-stimulated aloe leaves and a remedy from East Asian medicine has been developed; it has shown promising results with rheumatism, and by the criteria of academic medicine provides important findings concerning its working mechanism. It is a tea mixture from equal parts of

> dried bio-stimulated aloe leaves
> Tinnevelly-Sennes fruit,
> and leaves of Orthosiphones.

The Orthosiphones plant grows all over East Asia; in Indonesia it is of special quality. As a mono-drug, Orthosiphones is known in Europe as East Indian kidney tea. The leaves have a certain resemblance to peppermint. The pharmacology of the plant is noteworthy. In the course of animal experiments an Orthosiphones infusion increased the diuresis, as well as the excretion of chloride; in case of lead poisoning the excretion of lead. Glomerulo-filtration, i.e. natural rinsing of the kidneys, was considerably activated. Clinical examinations proved a good flushing-out of edemas in cases of kidney ailments and heart insufficiency. Orthosiphones stimulates gall bladder function and has a slightly spasmolytic effect.

Orthosiphones contains the valuable glycoside orthosiphonin, also the saponin sapophonin, essential oils and potassium salts.

Sennes fruit (pods) are very important for digestion, because rheumatic phenomena tend to go hand in hand with disturbances of intestinal activity. Sennes fruit promotes the detoxication of the organism. The loss of potassium through prolonged use of Senna is roughly balanced out by Orthosiphones. Aloe leaves, which have a slightly laxative effect, contain the necessary stimulants within their bio-stimulated active agents to mobilize the body's defenses via the central nervous system against the causes of rheumatic diseases.

This tea mixture must not be used during pregnancy and menstruation.

In order to increase the effect of the tea therapy we recommend a complementary therapy with aloe extract from bio-stimulated aloe leaves (watery extract): for the duration of one month, two weekly injections of 1 ml each are administered subcutaneously into the skin of the thigh. During the following injection-free phase of four weeks, the tea therapy is to be continued. After these four weeks, the cure should be repeated. Whereas the complete injection cure should be repeated only after one year, the tea therapy should be kept up for the duration of the disease, until a cure is effected. The tea prepared according to the enclosed instructions should be drunk twice a day, one cup each. Injected aloe extract decreases uric acid. This is one of the most important pre-conditions for a successful treatment of rheumatism.

In the long run, therapies of rheumatism can only bring success if the patient keeps a proper diet. Such a diet aims mainly at counteracting the formation of uric acid. Therefore all foods must be avoided which favor the formation of uric acid (purine). Amont these we find: pure coffee, black tea, cocoa, alcohol (including beer), chocolate, cakes and pastries, soup of all kinds, fish and smoked foods, salt, sugar, meat and sausages, jams and sweet dishes, lentils, peas, beans, cauliflower.

The above-mentioned foods are forbidden. Foods permitted: fresh fruit, potatoes, cottage cheese, fresh vegetables, camembert as well as other kinds of cheese low in salt, egg yolk, bread (whole wheat bread excepted), grains low in salt, vegetable fat, small amounts of noodles, nuts.

Especially to be recommended: red radishes, celery root, cucumbers, horse-radish, comfrey, cabbage, champignons, melons, lemons, and unsugared grape juice.

Thanks to international trade even the menu of a patient of rheumatism can be varied and appetizing. Also birch juice is recommended because it calms inflammations and flushes out uric acid, alternated with stinging-nettle juice, which stimulates the metabolism.

The recommended tea mixture is available in pharmacies and health-food stores.

MYELITIS

including polio

As aloe can now be counted among medicinal plants which most beneficently influence cell metabolism, the therapy with aloe extract is suitable for all those diseases in which cell tissue and nerve cells are afflicted.

Among these we count all those painful ailments which are denoted by the scientific term myelitis. The best-known among these is the fateful poliomyelitis, in short polio, which afflicts children. It is an acute inflammation of the anterior horn of the gray matter in the spinal marrow. The symptoms of the inflammation of the spinal marrow resemble the indications of multiple sclerosis.

The following therapy is recommended:

---

1. For grown-ups:

On 30 consecutive days one daily injection of 1 ml of aloe estract to be administered subcutaneously (thigh). After a 30-day interval, 30 more injections follow, one a day in the morning hours, to be followed by 15 to 20 minutes of rest.

If on some days severe pains should set in (primary deterioration), 0,5 ml of a 1 % novocain solution may be injected according to the doctor's specifications.

2. For children five years or older, in case of polio

On four consecutive days 0,5 ml each of aloe extract to be injected under the skin of the thigh; from the 5th through the 25th injection the above amount is to be injected only every other day. After 28 injection-free days of rest, eight more injections of 0,5 ml each follow at daily intervals. After another seven days of rest without injections, the cure is completed with a series of altogether 14 injections of 0,5 ml each, to be administered subcutaneously every other day. These are rather general recommendations, which can be modified by the attending doctor.

As long as the patient has a temperature, he should fast. Nutrition should consist only of pure cherry juice. As soon as the fever is gone, the diet should consist of fruit and raw vegetables. The back, including the small of the back, should be massaged with olive oil frequently (four times a day).

The causes are usually serious infectious diseases such as measles, rubella, typhoid fever, malaria, pneumonia; the disease can also be triggered by germs carried in the blood stream. As we can see, it is essential that these basic ailments are treated properly and cured.

In his experiments with spinal marrow, Prof. Barsegjan noted after an aloe injection cure that there was a »strengthening of regenerative processes«, among others the **restoration of impulse conduction across the bisected section of spinal marrow!**

SCHIZOPHRENIA

This often inconspicuous, severe ailment is an endogenic psychosis, i.e. not triggered by outside influences, but developing in the organism itself. According to the classic medical dictionary, PSCHYREMBEL, its cause is unknown.

Shortly before his death in 1936, the world-famous Russian psychologist Pavlov, who for many years had concerned himself with the problems of schizophrenia, stated the following:

»In the process of experimental diseases of the central nervous system, several indications of hypnosis tend to appear, as a sign of the physiological battle against the cause of the disease. Therefore the catatonic form of schizophrenia (i.e. one which progresses in connection with abnormal phases of excitement) with its hypnotic symptoms can be seen as a physiological, protective inhibition, which restricts the activity of the diseased brain and eventually eliminates it completely. So the first therapeutic measure should be setting it at rest.

Therefore in Pavlov's clinics the sleep therapy was especially popular.

Schizophrenia is characterized by a disturbance of the thinking process. The patient develops a peculiar, unreal logic, his relationship to his immediate surroundings is disturbed, he experiences the world in a changed manner, the meaning of every-day information and experiences is altered ominously and seen in correlation with himself; telvision news, for example, reporting problems of some kind are seen as coded warnings directed at the patient himself; the meaning of words within the thinking process is altered, with blockages, denial, and inspirations playing a part. Finally the derangement of thinking leads to total collapse. The patient's temperament is changed considerably: on the one hand there are erratic phases of irritability; on the other hand there are times of complete passivity, then again boisterous spells and aggressiveness. Hallucinations are common.

In the West, schizophrenia is treated by chemotherapy in combination with shock therapy and psycho-social methods, i.e. work therapies, social stimulation of the patient.

As stated above, curative sleep is one of the bases of Pavlov's therapy. In his analysis on sleep treatment and other therapies, Dr. Max Brandt adds:

»Special emphasis ought to be placed on the methods of conditionally reflective sleep, treatment with suggested sleep and the use of hypnosis, with which a sufficiently deep and long sleep can be effected and at the same time the use of barbiturates decreased.

12 to 15 days are recommended as the duration of sleep treatment in cases of chronic endogenic or nervous afflictions. A one-day interval in the middle is advisable. The duration of the treatment should be individually timed for each patient, depending on his condition and the character of his affliction. The patient should be awakened gradually. Two days before the completion of the sleep therapy the daily dose of barbiturates should be reduced by degrees (to about half). One or two days after the barbiturates are discontinued, the patient is transferred from his single room to the communal room. During the final stages of sleep therapy the patient needs special care and observation. During this period he should receive an ample amount of beverages, baths and intravenous application of glucose with ascorbic acid and thiamine. The treatment with various methods based on the principle of protective inhibition does not preclude the use of other healing compounds and therapeutic measures which are suited to the character of the patient's disease.«

We are of the opinion that sleep therapy can only effect the basic precondition, i.e. a position of rest, with strict attention to be paid to counter-indications: during extended sleep it is possible that irrational processes among the activities of the higher nerves of the patient are stronger than the inhibitory processes.

Therefore it is advisable to look out for biological therapy methods which can positively influence the course of the disease without harmful side-effects.

Tissue therapy was tried in the case of schizophrenia.

The Research Institute for Psychiatry in Moscow, for example, used tissue therapy on a broad scale. 43 patients with schizophrenia and 39 with traumatic psychoses showed good healing results. »Here too«, Dr. Max Brandt states, »tissue therapy as a method with non-specific healing effect has proved its mettle.«

It is important that this physician and researcher should be quoted on the subject. He is an expert on Soviet medicine and, where necessary, an uncompromising, even harsh critic. When schizophrenics were treated with the tissue therapy, better cures were noted in cases of slowly progressing, periodic deterioration, especially with patients showing abnormal excitability, and hypochondriacs. The successes in cases of psychoses of a traumatic nature (after injuries), however, were effected not only by means of the tissue therapy, but also by a combination with other therapies (insulin, deep sleep). Among a »multitude of organic and functional ailments of the nervous system«, Dr. Max Brandt names a few: »Through the implantation of segments from spleen, testicles, and thyroid glands the number of epileptic seizures could be reduced.«

Since the school of Filatow progressed from the implantation method of tissue therapy to a preponderant use of the aloe therapy, the injection method with aloe extract has been used with schizophrenia as well as with epilepsy. The author recommends the following therapy to the attending doctors:

After putting the patient into a position of rest and in harmony with psychological measures:

On 25 consecutive days one daily ampulla of 1 ml of aloe extract to be injected subcutaneously into the thigh. During an injection-free pause of 30 days the other therapies continue unchanged. Another cure phase of 30 injections at daily intervals follows, application as above.

This cure is to be repeated three times at yearly intervals. If actual or simulated pains appear, the cure should be interrupted for three days and the daily dosage of the injection reduced to 0,5 ml.

In the recent past reliable reports of successes in the treatment of this severe, malignant disease have become known.

SCLERODERMIA (HARDENING OF THE SKIN)

At an advanced stage this disease is a serious, often deadly system disease (Pschyrembel). It is characterized by indications of deficit: lack of minerals, deficient gland activity, disturbance of the vessel system up to the point of vessel atrophy. Deficiency symptoms are accompanied by growths of connective tissues and atrophy of the skin. Fingers and toes become stiff or circulation in them is constricted. Typical phenomena are the so-called »Madonna fingers« and the »mask face«. Other symptoms of this disease are wounds that are difficult to heal. In many cases interior organs are affected: esophagus (swallowing difficulties), nephrosclerosis, myocardsclerosis.

Academic medicine has no adequate therapy to offer.

Physiomedicine (Dr. Brauchle) offers air baths, sun baths, increased raw vegetarian diet as well as remedial gymnastics in hot water. All this is absolutely correct as it causes the disease to stagnate.

Now the aloe-extract therapy, tried out in many exacting clinical tests, offers the first prospect of a cure. It is applied as follows:

On 30 consecutive days, one ampulla of 1 ml of aloe extract each is injected subcutaneously in the morning hours. After an interval of rest of another 30 days the second therapy phase follows, comprising 30 more injections, i.e. every day one injection of 1 ml under the skin (thigh). After one year the cure should be repeated. The biogenic stimulators of the aloe remedy the deficiencies and strengthen the immune system.

RADIATION INJURIES

The blessings of X-ray treatment as well as the whole system of modern therapies including ray treatment unfortunately can exact a high price: severe damages and burns of the skin, malignant abscesses, ulcers and tissue inflammations. Frequently swellings also develop.

In all known cases the therapy with aloe compounds has brought about lasting cures. It seems like an omen that in our epoch, which is marked by growing fear of the devastating consequences of ray-treatment injuries, a system of active agents can be proved to exist in the aloe, the Biblical plant, which offers protection against, and cure of, radiation injuries. As this discovery is of utmost importance in medical history we would like to give a convincing report about the program »aloe against radiation injuries«:

In the laboratory the influence of an emulsion from bio-stimulated aloe juice on the chronological progress of radiation injuries in the skin of rabbits was examined. Skin damage through radiation is effected by radioactive phosphorus in the form of a flat applicator being fastened to the shaved area. The dosage used was 6000 r. After removal of the applicator, aloe emulsion was applied twice a day for 12 consecutive days. With another group of rabbits, the skin areas were treated with an ointment containing no aloe extract; a third group was not treated at all. The skin areas treated with aloe emulsion developed a temporary redness. After three days the skin started flaking off, which lasted for eight days. During this period the skin became elastic and turned pink; new fur started growing. With the group not treated with aloe extract, on the first days after the applicator was removed a swelling of the skin was observed. After four days the skin started flaking off, too. After six days a moist epidermis started forming, which turned into a yellowish-reddish crust that fell off after 15 days. The skin regained its normal appearance, but no fur started growing.

With the rabbits treated with aloe, the healing of the skin took 12 days; with the control group without an aloe treatment it took 21 days.

Thereupon the aloe emulsion underwent numerous tests in the X-ray and radiology institute. They were clinical observations of patients who had undergone radiation therapy and suffered malignant side-effects in their skin. Exterior radiation methods had been used. Depending on the afflicted place of swelling, face, chest and groin were examined.

The first group of 90 test patients received aloe-emulsion treatment prior to radiation. This emulsion was thinly applied to the test areas. In those cases where after radiation, but before the use of aloe, a skin reaction was noted, aloe emulsion was applied every other day up to the end of the treatment.

The second group of 90 control patients received no aloe emulsion. Instead other ointments were used. Patients with analogical indications were observed, and local radiation was administered. Out of the 90 test patients treated with aloe, 38 showed no skin reactions. 30 test patients noted a very short-term reddening. With these patients the radiation dosage could be 1000 r higher than with the control group. Only 22 test patients developed the moist epidermis after a radiation dose of 4500 to 6000 r. In contrast, all patients of the control group developed this symptom at a dosage of 3500 r.

These findings make it imperative that the aloe compounds be placed in the hands of every radiologist as well as clinician concerned with radiation treatment and radiation injuries.

---

1. **Prior to X-ray examinations:** Aloe emulsion should be lightly applied to the areas to be examined.

2. In case of radiation injuries in the realm of Beta-UV, of burns, of sunburn and for treating malignant abscesses, aloe emulsion is to be applied to the afflicted areas twice a day for 12 consecutive days. In more complicated cases aloe syrup should be taken in addition, one teaspoon twice or three times a day at mealtimes for 10 days.

As a protection against the sun, and thus a prophylactic measure against sunburn, aloe cream can be recommended. It is important that only creams expressly denoted as bio-stimulated are used. Those creams currently on the market named »ALOE-Vera« are not bio-stimulated. In addition the bio-stimulated creams have a constringent effect. Thus a plant thousands of years old bares only now its profoundest secret from the wisdom of creation and gives the people of the age of radiation the first real hope.

DUODENAL ULCERS

The so-called duodenalulcera can pose serious problems to the afflicted person, especially the one who consults his doctor too late in the false belief that he has gastric ulcers and therefore reacts wrongly. Duodenal ulcers afflict the male sex more frequently than the female one. In case of both gastric and duodenal ulcers blood appears in the stool, and gastric juice is hyperacid. Only an X-ray examination can pinpoint the location of the ulcer (do not forget to apply aloe emulsion before the examination as a protection against X-rays! Cf. the chapter on radiation injuries). There is an effective biological therapy for duodenal ulcers:

Three times daily one teaspoon of bio-stimulated aloe juice to be taken after each meal, to be followed by a few small sips of milk.
This therapy should last between three weeks and, at most, two months.

In case of complications and at an advanced stage an injection cure with aloe extract should be started immediately:

For 30 consecutive days one daily injection of 1 ml to be given under the skin (thigh); after an injection-free phase of 30 days, the second cure phase with 30 injections of 1 ml each follows.

The therapy recommendations concerning aloe juice as well as aloe-extract injections that are given above also apply to enteritis, i.e. the inflammation of the small intestine, which has the same symptoms as gastritis.

ALOE AS USED IN POPULAR MEDICINE

For a long time medical practitioners in Polynesia and especially on Hawaii have known aloe to be a medicinal herb. According to travelers' reports, the natives of the South Sea islands used to crush the leaves to make a curative ointment for arthritis.

For wounds that are difficult to heal, popular medicine knows aloe compresses, i.e. aloe tincture diluted 1 to 10 is applied to the wounds, rubbed in lightly, and covered with a compress.

In cases of colon catarrh with the liver being also affected, taking a dilution of the homeopathic potency D-4 is common. As we know, academic medicine has made use of these practical experiences by prescribing aloe in the so-called galenical compounds, i.e. in the form of drops, pills, suppositories, injections and dragées as a reliable laxative. The reader should realize that these aloe preparations, both the ones from popular medicine and those available in the pharmacy are by no means the same things as the active agents of bio-stimulated aloe-tissue compounds. These compounds are absolutely new, they do not have a laxative influence, but have effects as described in the different chapters of this publication.

Russian and Asian popular medicine, especially in China and India, have known aloe preparations as a bitter stomach remedy which also improves gall secretion.

In the Cinese pharmacology of Li Shih-Shen (1518 — 1593) the aloe is repeatedly named as an important medicinal herb. It is an especially effective variety, Lu-huei or aloe chinensis. It is applied as a juice for the exterior treatment of wounds, as a tonic, for the treatment of ailments of the stomach and intestinal tract as an extract or in the form of pills.

It is noteworthy that aloe chinensis (sinensis Steud., a Chinese variety of the aloe) is also listed as one of the most important remedies against arteriosclerosis. This is all the more remarkable as this aloe extract is untreated, i.e. has not been bio-stimulated, which would have increased its effect considerably. The author has found traditional Chinese medicine to be absolutely reliable, including its pharmacological information. The doctors of ancient China used to give detailed prescriptions for the application of medicaments with regard to the time of day, position of the sun and phases of the moon. People in the West tended to dismiss this as astrological nonsense. Meanwhile modern biological research has shown up the fact that all living processes are subject to biological rhythms, which is to say that the healing intensity of drugs does vary according to the time of day, seasons, even the periods of sun spots.

East Indian medicine knows a whole series of applications of the local aloe variety, called kumari. Besides the leaves they even use the roots of the plant. One of the main areas of application is skin diseases, boils, abscesses, cysts, tumors and ulcers. Popular medicine has always known the invigorating effect of aloe on the whole organism. After all this turned out to be the starting point for Filatow on his way to tissue therapy.

The old Christian community at Edessa produced incense from the trunk of the aloe. To this incense they ascribed mystic powers of cleansing the soul. This might be in close correlation with the therapeutic use of aloe leaves and juices by the priest-doctors of antiquity. The scent emanating from the essential oils conveys the feeling of well-being and thus contains a religious component. The effect of the heavenly fragrance conveys closeness to God, and in the presence of the rising incense, the believer is cleansed of sin. This is certainly a magic principle, but from all we know it is based on curative experience with the plant. Orthodox churches have actively taken over the use of various scents and ointments; the correlation with the rites of the Old Testament is still evident. These fragrant plants have acquired their importance not only because they are used in holy rites, but also because of their God-given curative effect; their »Godly substances« make them worthy of being integrated into holy services. The liturgical books of the Orthodox churches give precise directions concerning the composition of aromatic substances as they are used in sacramental rites. There we find aloe at the top.

The active incorporation of aromatic substances into healing practice in the Orthodox churches is quite pronounced. There these substances not only convey spiritual blessings, but also curative and protective powers. Their scent is seen as a curative agent in the medical sense, with properties to ward off physical ailments, and a special prayer of consecration is used for aromatic herbs. The church of Edessa, which handed on its experience and religious principles to the famous theological school of Edessa, had learned the use of aromatic substances and healing agents directly from the apostle Judas Thaddaeus, who composed the letter in the New Testament named after him and who stayed in Edessa several times, moreover in Armenia, Persia and Aserbeidshan.

Undoubtedly this apostle had his medical knowledge, including the use of herbs, from Jesus Christ himself, who in his turn had probably acquired his practical healing knowledge from the secret sect of the Essener before taking up his public vocation. Finds of papyrus scrolls and recent discoveries in the manuscripts of the Monastery of St. Catherine on Sinai indicate that the Essener sect had a complete knowledge of healing.

It is interesting to note that in several East Asian religions aloe wood is burned in liturgic rites and that the fragrance thereof is seen as a mystic healing and cleansing agent to be used as a protection against demons. The reputation of the aloe as a »holy plant« also reached the priest Sebastian Kneipp. He investigated the traditions and used aloe successfully in pediatrics, mainly with eye afflictions. He had the eyes rinsed daily with water containing some diluted aloe.

Moreover we find aloe mentioned in old medical manuscripts dealing with Swedish herbs and Swedish bitters.

In view of the results of modern research it becomes understandable that the powers of life contained in this medicinal herb are seen as a special part of creation.

THE METHOD OF BIO-STIMULATION

Freshly cut aloe leaves are washed with water and kept in a dark room at a temperature of 6° to 8° C for 12 to 15 days.

Within the tissues of the aloe, active compounds now organize themselves into bio-stimulators. The juice extracted from the residue is again kept at 6° C in darkness for about 12 days, then the treatment is continued with a certain procedure.

The chapter on the aloe healing system describes at great length how the preconditions for the formation of biogenic stimulators are created and **how the biogenic stimulators can be proved**.

To preclude misunderstandings we would like to point out the following: the German Homeopathic Book of Medicine (Deutsches Homöopathisches Arzneibuch) in prescription number 38 deals with the production of watery basic tinctures by treatment with cold, and with their liquid dilutions. The prescription runs as follows:

»The finely chopped plant material is put into a solution six times its own quantity, which consists of 8,8 parts of sodium chloride, 0,2 parts of sodium-hydrogen carbonate, and 991 parts of water (for injection purposes: aqua ad injectabilia).

This mixture is stored at a temperature of about 4° C for 14 days, being stirred mornings and evenings. Afterwards the juice is pressed out and kept at about 4° C, protected from light, until it has turned completely clear. This remaining clear basic tincture undergoes further treatment immediately.«

In the case of the aloe this procedure leads only to a laxative. There is no bio-stimulation. Bio-stimulation takes place in the leaves, or better, in their tissue. Therefore the above-quoted prescription number 38 should not create the erroneous assumption that it is the treatment of the tinctures by cold and darkness, which creates the biogenic stimulators. The process for the leaves cut off from the stem whose tissues organize their survival, is absolutely new and follows the laws of organic life, not only those of homeopathy. For Western academic medicine, this work with biogenic stimulators in connection with the indications listed in this publication is completely new.

ON THE BOTANY OF THE ALOE

The aloe belongs to the liliaceae, i.e. to the family of the lilies. The perennially green plant is also called »century plant«.

The leaves grow in successive order and are fleshy and juicy. The blossoms grow in clusters; with many kinds of aloe they are orange, but colors vary. The fruit is shaped like a tiny cylindrical box. The plant grows like a tree with a maximum height of 20 feet. The main harvest time is between the end of October and the end of November. Only the leaves are harvested. Aloe trees originated in southern Africa. Synonyms are African aloe (aloe ferox), Socotra aloe (aloe perryi), »aloe« in German and Russian, »aloes« in French, »kumari« in Hindi, and »Lu-huei« in Chinese.

The aloe is at home in Africa, it is grown in South and East Africa; this is the Cape aloe. Furthermore it is planted in some states of the American continent, in the West Indies and in coastal areas of Venezuela. This variety is called Curacao aloe, because traditionally the plant is exported from this port. It is also called Barbados aloe. Aloe arborescens is cultivated in the USSR, in Turkey, Israel, India and China. Moreover it is to be found in southern Italy and Greece, on Cyprus, in Spain and Portugal, in Arab countries as well as the South Sea.

Some names were coined by traders according to places of origin: Uganda aloe, Natal aloe, Zanzibar aloe, Cape aloe (aloe capensis), Socotra aloe, and finally Mocca aloe, which reminds us of the classic land of the Queen of Sheba.

Mocca and Socotra aloe are known to have an especially high content of active agents. Already the apostle Thomas, himself well-versed in antique medicine, came to know the aloe on the Yemenitic Isle of Sokotra. On his way from Palestine, Thomas stayed there in A.D. 52 to prepare for his Indian mission. With the merchant Habban, who did business in the Arab world in the service of the Indian king Gondophar, the apostle first traveled to Cranganore on the Malabar Coast — today this is the Indian state of Kerala. Under the protection of the Hindu kings St. Thomas did missionary work in the name of Jesus Christ and healed the sick. His knowledge concerning the healing agents of the aloe, especially in the treatment of wounds, was of great advantage to him. In those days, which were marked by bloody wars, healing wounds was a task of eminent importance, same as the treatment of ulcers, which on account of poor hygiene spread rapidly in the hot regions. In this way one of the greatest figures of the New Testament introduced an ancient medicinal herb in India, where it is still playing an essential role within the framework of medical services; nowadays its importance is also scientifically proved.

The botany of the more than 250 aloe varieties throughout the world has by far not been completely researched. As becomes evident from the story of the apostle Thomas, the aloe is not without reason mentioned in the Old Testament, and through the latest research in our times has bared many secrets for the good of mankind — but we can surely expect more surprises when other varieties are examined, such as the Mocca aloe, whose chemistry is practically unknown. A research grant in this direction would be a lot more meaningful than many a space-exploration series, not only in the material sense, but also therapeutically and ethically.

ON THE CHEMISTRY OF THE ALOE

A scientific treatise on the complete chemistry of the plant would go beyond the bounds of a therapy handbook of popular science. Therefore we will state only a few principal facts. Those interested in in-depth information can write for more material to the address of the research group listed on page 6.

For the production of laxatives, which is not the subject of this publication, all varieties of the aloe are suited. Aloe which is not bio-stimulated is generally known as a laxative.

For the procedure of bio-stimulation all kinds of Curacao aloe are not suited as they contain no aloisides, which are indispensable for the working mechanism of the biogenic stimulators. Cape aloe, however, aloe arborescens, Socotra, Natal, and Uganda aloe do contain aloisides. With Mocca aloe we do not yet know. According to recent research, varieties without aloisides can also be found among the Cape aloes. At present we do not know any reason for the appearance of two Cape varieties. As the drug is produced by the same process and other influences can be discounted, we may presume that chemically differentiated variants of aloe ferox exist and are used for production.

The aloe leaves contain aloe-emodin, aloin, more precisely barb-aloin, the aloisides A and B (in varying proportions), chromon derivatives, also so-called aloesines and amaroids such as aloenin.

There are aloe varieties containing up to 18 % of aloisides. Far more than twenty different components have been proved to exist in the aloe, among them those organic acids separately described in connection with the biogenic stimulators, which correspond with the citric-acid cycle in the human organism. The chain of barb-aloin, aloesin, aloenin and the aloisides A und B from bio-stimulated aloe tissues form the biochemical structure which corresponds to the finely structured, high-molecular substances of the information conduction of the central nervous system.

THE »HOMEOPATHIC EFFECT« OF THE ALOE THERAPY

The aloe-injection solution consists of 1% of watery basic tincture and of 99% of water as aqua ad iniectabilia. In this composition the injection is administered by the physicians. In homeopathic terms this composition can be expressed by: D 2. This denotes the second potency, i.e. the second homeopathic dilution level. The success of the aloe therapy in this dilution allows a conclusion concerning the effectiveness of homeopathic potencies as a whole. Of course we must concede that the effectiveness of aloe extract, even in weaker dilutions, must be ascribed to the biogenic stimulators. Nevertheless the aloe experiment points a way for homeopathy in its struggle for a scientific proof of its effect, which it has sought to establish since its beginning. It has been proved that the aloe injection takes effect via the central nervous system, with its influence on the activity of the cerebral enzyme systems being of particular importance. The biogenic stimulators from the aloe affect those receptors or »command posts« which program and run the healthy organism and its defense system against disease. As we can see, this mechanism is set in motion by a system of signals. With the aloe it is the biogenic stimulators which trigger this signal effect. In all homeopathic preparations of high potency, it is the high-molecular, finely structured substances which through their signals to the central nervous system activate the switches corresponding to the organs concerned; in the same way as with the biogenic stimulators they may provide minute information material, as far as deficits thereof exist, and ultimately they may trigger a re-programming in the direction of healing activities.

If these findings are correct, future homeopathy should be divided into two categories: the material homeopathy up to a dilution or comminution level of D 6, and high-potency homeopathy. In homeopathical practice the adherents of high-potency therapy diverge so radically from the adherents of low-potency therapy that such a division would be warranted.

In low-potency homeopathy the substances used are still of measurable quantities, whereas the adherents of high-potency homeopathy claim that it works »spiritually«, in a higher mental realm. Here they state something that is correct, but with their somewhat nebulous explanation they hand arguments to the opponents of homeopathy, who use them to dismiss successful homeopathic cures as placebo effects. This amounts to maintaining that homeopathic preparations are pseudo-medicaments, which is both grotesque and irresponsible, as placebo effects are scientifically even less researched than homeopathy. Most opponents of homeopathy can be considered incompetent judges because they have not investigated homeopathy scientifically. The causes of these misjudgements are to be found in the scientific bondage to categories of quantity rather than quality. Calling for a scientific proof of the effect of homeopathy diverts attention from the impotency of established science to deal with homeopathy in a scientific manner. At the same time this restricts the patient's freedom to choose a certain therapy; what he seeks above all is being cured, not scientific treatment which often trades one disease with the side-effects of another. Our knowledge from the aloe therapy, i.e. that high-potency homeopathy constitutes a signal system for the central nervous system, ought to pave the way towards proving the effect according to scientific criteria. After all homeopathy works in a scientific way: it involves diagnosis and anamnesis as well as a prognosis as to the course of the disease, healing and control-examinations. Moreover it need not restrict itself to animal experiments, but has an experience of more than 200 years from working with human patients, where in cases of analogical symptoms the therapy differentiates between different constitutional types of the patients and their disposition for a certain disease.

In view of this knowledge man will become aware that as a being to be treated in its totality he is an ecological part of a nature-organism, through which and in accordance to which he functions. Health and disease are defined according to this awareness. If he realizes that he can remedy deficits from other systems of life such as plants, minerals and other healing agents, he will easily get well; if however through ignorance he violates the ecological concept of health, he will be treated, but by no means cured!

INGREDIENTS AND RECIPES FOR COMPOUNDS TO BE USED IN THE ALOE HEALING SYSTEM

1. Aloe-injection solution

The aloe-injection solution consists of a watery basic tincture from the bio-stimulated juice extracted from fresh leaves of aloe capensis.

It is produced according to special prescriptions in accordance with the Homöopathisches Arzneibuch (Book of Homeopathic Medicaments) of the German Federal Republic.

Ascorbic-phosphate buffer solution is used as the carrier of healing compounds. The watery basic tincture is diluted to the homeopathic potency of D 2.

This production is permitted only to licensed pharmaceutical companies in possession of the requried patents in accordance with pharmaceutical law.

2. Pressed aloe juice (succus aloes)

80 ml of watery solution from the juice of fresh aloe leaves (aloe ferox Mill.; for bio-stimulation the leaves are previously stored in a cool, dark room for 12 to 14 days.)

20 ml of ethanol 95 % proof

The leaves must be washed carefully in hot water.

Afterwards they are finely chopped, wrapped in gauze and pressed.

The resulting suspension is filtered. This is carried out using mull (if necessary under pressure).

The filtred juice is heated to the boiling point for 8 to 10 minutes, then poured into a clarifying container. Now the necessary quantity of ethanol is added. This mixture is stored in a cool, dark place and stirred once a day. Afterwards it is filtered finely once again.

3. Ferruginous pressed aloe juice (succus aloes cum ferro)

This special juice for the treatment of anemia has a composition as follows:

14,3 parts of bio-stimulated plant material, 0,15 parts of haematite, 50,0 parts of purified water (»Ampuwa«, sterile aqua ad iniectabilia free of pyrogenic substances)

In the morning this mixture is placed into a water bath of about 37° C. In the evening the mixture is placed into water containing ice, to be stirred immediately before and after this procedure. Then the mixture is again placed into a water bath of 37° C. After 24 more hours the juice is pressed out. After several hours it is filtered through mull. As a rule the filtered liquid is turgid.

4. Ferruginous aloe syrup (sirupus aloes cum ferro)

One part of the juice produced according to the directions above (chapter 3) is boiled with one part of sugar and immediately filled into brown glass bottles.

5. Aloe emulsion (emulsum aloes)

For 100 grammes of aloe emulsion one needs:

70 gr of watery solution from the bio-stimulated fresh juice of aloe leaves (all varieties except aloe barbadensis and aloes free of aloisides), 15 gr of castor oil, 15 gr of emulgator (ketyl alcohol or lecithin), 0,1 gr of eucalyptus oil.

The first three components are mixed together, heated in a water bath and stirred until completely homogenized. Finally the eucalyptus oil is added, and the mixture stirred until cold.

6. Aloe skin-protection cream

Composition:

6 grammes of beeswax (white), 6 gr of walrat, 40 gr of sweet almond oil, 20 gr of watery aloe tincture D 1 from bio-stimulated aloe leaves (all varieties except aloe capensis and varieties free of aloisides)

THE AGAVE HEALING SYSTEM

Tissue therapy, the aloe healing system and the agave therapy form a scientific unit because all three are characterized by the biogenic stimulators, which unfold their healing powers; besides they have in common that they are non-specific stimulation therapies.

The agave – agava americana – is for the first time introduced into the medical practice of Western Europe by the ARBEITSGEMEINSCHAFT GRUNDLAGENFORSCHUNG FÜR BIOLOGISCHE MEDIZIN, i.e. through this publication.

It is not contained in any official book of medicaments of the West, even though its long-lasting use in popular medicine should have been stimulation enough to examine its active agents. But it may well be true that certain circles consider it irrelevant whether an inexpensive biological remedy which nature grants us is given preference over expensive chemotherapy. Responsible doctors, however, will always make use of knowledge which offers new prospects of healing for their patients. Prof. Filatow M. D., oculist of world-renown (see previous chapters), found it worth his while to examine the treasure trove of popular medicine in order to make use of medicinal herbs for the benefit of modern medicine. He was the first one to examine the agave in a scientific way. Popular medicine in the Caucasus has for a long time known the root and the leaves of the agave as a remedy against tuberculosis. This is where Filatow continued with his research. In experiments he proved that the extract from agava americana, same as aloe extract, heals tuberculosis of the skin. In pharmacological experiments he noted that the juice from young agave leaves has a diuretic and laxative effect. Thus we have an important, entirely natural remedy, which rinses the urinary passages and has a mild laxative effect, and at the same time invigorates the organism by its stimulating qualities! The agave contains the sugar agavose ($C_{12}H_{22}O_{11}$) as well as resins and saponins. Filatow stated that in the tissues of the agave, same as with the aloe, active agents of an »undefined nature« develop if the leaves are preserved in cold and darkness. Evidently this is also a case of biogenic stimulators at work.

Based on clinical experience a considerable amount of literature on the agave therapy has been written in Russia. As early as 1950 a scientific treatise on the biological activity of the extracts from conserved agave leaves was published in Kiev. Later on medical institutes published reports about the treatment of complicated eye diseases with agave extracts and about the effects of a watery agave extract on stomach secretion. This is a field of experience of popular medicine already known to Mexican as well as ancient Aztec practice. The agave is cultivated not only in sub-tropical regions of Georgia (Caucasus), Abchasia and on the Crimea, but also in its countries of origin, Mexico and South America. In 1561 the agave was introduced into Europe by the Spanish Conquistadors, first to Spain, Portugal, Italy, southern France, southern Turkey, and even into the Swiss canton of Ticino. The agave belongs to the family of narcissus plants. Because of their juice rich in sugar some varieties of the agave have long been used as food. Shortly before flowering time, the juice is pressed from the bloom. It contains 9 to 10 % cane sugar and 2,5 % fructose. The Mexicans boil the juice down to a syrup, which is then dried into veritable loaves of sugar.

In Mexico the bluish-green agaves that grow as tall as a man are of special importance. Eight to ten years must pass until the centerpiece of the so-called blue agave has reached the right size for harvesting. This centerpiece is called Pina, and in its maturity resembles a pineapple. The juice of the Pina is the basis for healing remedies as well as for alcoholic products. The centerpiece of the blue agave yields about two litres (half a gallon). The Pina is as large as a pumpkin.

The native Indians of Mexico used the agave for healing purposes. Shortly before flowering time honey water is extracted from the centerpiece to be used for soothing and healing the stomach. The leaves are used as food, partly also as animal fodder.

Sometimes the sugary juice is fermented into a beverage similar to wine. After distillation, Mexicans drink it as herb brandy, as stomach brandy. Its soothing effect on the stomach is based on the important ferment papain, which enhances the digestion of protein. Here we do not want to recommend the brandy, but the juice from the agava americana as a stomach remedy. Agave juice is especially advisable in case of digestive troubles and heart burn. It should be taken after meals. Papain is also contained in the melon variety papaya and is a very important healing remedy. In view of the manifold curative agents contained in the agave, it constitutes a whole healing system. Through the process of bio-stimulation, the healing powers are increased, as stated and proved in the chapter on the aloe.

Another remark concerning papain: it is an enzyme which improves digestion and rejuvenates the digestive system. The working mechanism of papain constitutes a kind of breathing aid as it eliminates heavy mucus in the respiratory ducts and soothes coughing. Papain, being a protein-splitting enzyme, is able to heal wounds quickly by reducing degenerated proteins in the wounds. In American field hospitals papain preparations have within one week brought about complete healing of ulcers, muscle ailments and bed sores.

On account of their papain content, agave ointments aid in the dissolution of accumulated secretion in the pores. The agave ointment eliminates infectious waste material, cleans out the pores filled with sebaceous matter, increases body respiration and enhances youthful skin. Therefore preparations from the agave can be recommended as a scalp embrocation against seborrhoea.

According to proven scientific experience, agave juice is to be applied (taking into account what we know about the development of biogenic stimulators) in the following cases:

1. Recuperation processes after serious diseases, on account of its invigorating properties concerning vitality
2. Inflammations, and for cleansing the urinary passages and the kidneys in the diuretic sense
3. For digestive troubles, heart burn, gastritis, for strengthening the stomach, especially the gastric membranes in connection with the enzyme papain, which effects a rejuvenation of the digestive system
4. For bronchial coughs, for eliminating mucus from the respiratory tract, again on account of its papain content
5. For healing wounds, as papain reduces degenerated proteins in the wounds.

Using the juice as a cure means taking it pure without sugar added, to be drunk by the patient at a dosage of one wine glass of agave juice two or three times a day with meals.

Diabetics planning a cure with agave juice must consult their doctor for co-ordinating their whole diet plan concerning the intake of sugar; after all agave juice contains almost 10% cane sugar, and fructose besides.

For treating external wounds, papain powder from the agave is applied to the wounds and bed sores three times a day.

Embrocations with agave ointment for skin care and cleansing are applied twice a day, in the morning and in the evening hours. For treating seborrhoea, the ointment is applied four times a day and massaged in lightly.

For the extraction of curative and protective agents from the agave not only agava americana is suited, but also the varieties agava atrivirens and agava cantale.

INDEX OF DISEASES

FOREIGN WORDS AND MEDICAL TERMS

Adrenalin	a hormone produced by the suprarenal marrow, has a stimulating effect (increases blood pressure) — adrenalin is relased from the suprarenal marrow into the bloodstream through nervous impulses
Allopathy	a term coined by Samuel Hahnemann (founder of homeopathy) for academic medicine, i.e. the curative method in contrast to homeopathy
Analgesia	pain-stilling medicine
Anthroposophic medicine	procedure founded by Rudolf Steiner with naturally developed healing remedies being used to treat an organ in connection with the whole organism and to influence principal functions of life in their totality of body and soul
Antispasmodic	cramp relaxing
Application	to be applied, administered
Arresting	arrest = to nip a disease in the bud or to shorten the course of the illness greatly
Asthenia	feebleness, debility
Barbiturates	salts from barbituric acid, a basic substance of many sleeping pills
Brain capillaries	smallest blood vessels in the brain
Cerebral	having to do with the brain
Chill aetiology	aetiologies = doctrines of the causes of illness, in this case of chills.
Cholinesterase	splits acetylcholine into acetic acid and choline-acetylcholine, transmits nerve impulses from one nerve to another or to the various organs (the suppression of the cholinesterase has a soothing effect on the nerves)
Co-desmone system	a system of antibodies produced by biogenic stimulators
Co-enzyme system	Co-enzymes are substances which take part in enzyme reactions in which molecules are transmitted. They not only take up these molecules, but also release them again. Co-enzymes appear alone and also attached to enzymes. The combined action of different enzyme reactions, e.g. through biogenic stimulators, can be defined as a co-enzyme system.
Dehydrase, dehydrogenase	enzymes which belong to the so-called oxidoreductases. They split hydrogen from substrates (e.g. succinic acid, malic acid). The hydrogen, which is activated by the dehydrases is absorbed by the co-enzymes of cellular oxidation (respiratory chain) or is used in biosynthesis. This process releases energy.
Desmones	biogenic stimulators which can be compared to the cerebral-enzyme system and which stimulate this system
Dialectic medicine	Originally, dialectic is the art of uncovering inconsistencies through discussion and contradiction and getting to the bottom of the truth. Hegel defines dialectic as a movement of logic, which is characterized by a sequence of thesis — antithesis — synthesis. This philosophical term was first applied to medicine by Wirth. It

means integrating curative methods based on experience into academic medicine after an examination of their therapy results. According to this thesis, no curative method with proven effect should be disclaimed for the sole reason that academic medicine is as yet incapable of providing suitable testing methods to establish »proofs of effectiveness«. As a matter of principle, dialectic medicine does not see truth in a dialectic sense as being identical with the temporary truth of a scientific reality which can be made obsolete any time, which keeps changing, progressing. It is in the interest of medicine's highest aim, i.e. preventing and healing, to give precedence to the truth derived from verifiable cures of medicine based on experience over the limited truth of conservative testing methods and testing claims.

Dialysis	artificial rinsing of the kidneys by medical apparatus
Dilution	making weaker by mixing, a way of administering homeopathical remedies
Discogenic	coming from the interarticular disk
Diuresis	discharge or passing of urine
Diuretic	stimulating the release of urine
Endocrine glands	ductless glands of internal secretion, which secrete hormones directly into the bloodstream and lymphatic system, respectively (in contrast to the »exocrine glands« – external secretion – skin, mucous membranes)
Enzymes	high molecular protein substances which are produced in living cells (human, animal and plant). They are biocatalysts, i.e. they do not change the balance of a reaction but decrease the activation energy belonging to it. All enzymes belong chemically to the proteins or proteids (according to Pschyrembel). Active agents such as hormones or the biogenic stimulators regulate the biosynthesis through enzyme activity. That means that the regulation of the metabolism through enzymes takes place in accordance with superior controlling principles.
Geriatrics	medical science of old age
Glomerulo filtration	the natural cleansing of the blood through the kidneys
Glucose	grape sugar, to be found in the urine in cases of diabetes mellitus
Glutamic acid dehydrogenase	an enzyme which causes the conversion of the amino group to pyruvic acid (important intermediate product in carbohydrate metabolism = conversion of fats)
Glycerophosphate dehydrogenase	oxidation enzyme
Hemodynamic	examination of the blood circulation from the physical aspect (pressure, volume, flow, elasticity etc.)
Heteroglycanes	antibodies produced by biogenic stimulators
Hexenal sleep	short sleep induced by narcotics
Histological	concerning tissue; histology is the medical science of tissue
Hypothalamus	neurovegetative regulation center located beneath the thalamus, part of the mid-brain
Insufficiency	weak, inadequate power
Intoxication	toxicosis, serious course of diseases caused by poison
Ischemia	individual parts of organs are bloodless due to a deficient blood supply
Laxative	purgative
Locomotorial functions	functions referring to the locomotion of various functions

Lumbarsacral radiculitis	neuritis of the nerve roots in the lumbar vertebral and sacral area
Metabolism	the process by which food is built up into living matter or by which living matter is broken down into simple substances
Myopia	short-sightedness
Neurasthenia	This denotes the neurasthenic syndrome, i.e. the concurrence of abnormal irritability of the psychic functions and abnormal exhaustion
Orthosiphones	East Indian kidney tea
Oxidation enzymes	enzymes which transmit oxygen (significant for metabolism)
Pathogenesis	origin of disease
Potentiate	homeopathical dilution or grinding down (the designation D 6 shows for example the homeopathical power of a medicament, i.e. how much it has been diluted or ground down)
Remittence	temporary improvement of pathological symptoms
Resorption	absorption of substances into the blood and lymph paths
Sclera	outermost sturdy sheath covering the eye ball
Signature lore	Simon de Cordo published the first dictionary of signature lore in 1330. He explained the curative effect of plants through their color signals and symbolic forms (yellow flowers for liver and gall etc.)
Subcortical	below the cerebral cortex
Succinodehydrase, Succinathydrogenase	important enzyme in the citric acid cycle, converts succinic acid into maleic acid through dehydrogenization (splitting hydrogen); maleic acid is an oxidation product of human and also vegetable metabolism.
Succinoxydase, Succino	belonging to the group of oxidation enzymes
Sympathetic system	part of the nervous vegetative system
Thalamus	central subcortical collecting point and control station for all the sensitive and sensory stimuli from the environment and inner life flowing to the cerebrum, »door to consciousness«.
Thiamine	vitamine B1, influences cells that use a large amount of carbohydrates (nerve cells). Deficiency symptoms lead to serious diseases of the central nervous system.
Vascular (angio) spasms	vessel spasms
Vasomotorial, Vasculomotorial	concerning the vascular nerves
Vasotonia, tonus	elasticity of the blood vessels and the fine muscles that surround them
Vegetative dystonia	defective reaction of the nervous vegetative system consisting of the nervus vagus (tenth cerebral nerve) and the nervus sympathicus with functional disturbances of various organs
Yellow macule	place on the retina where sight is sharpest (yellow spot on the retina of the eye)
Zytochromoxydase	belonging to the oxidation enzymes that transmit oxygen and in this way effect an oxidation of the metabolism

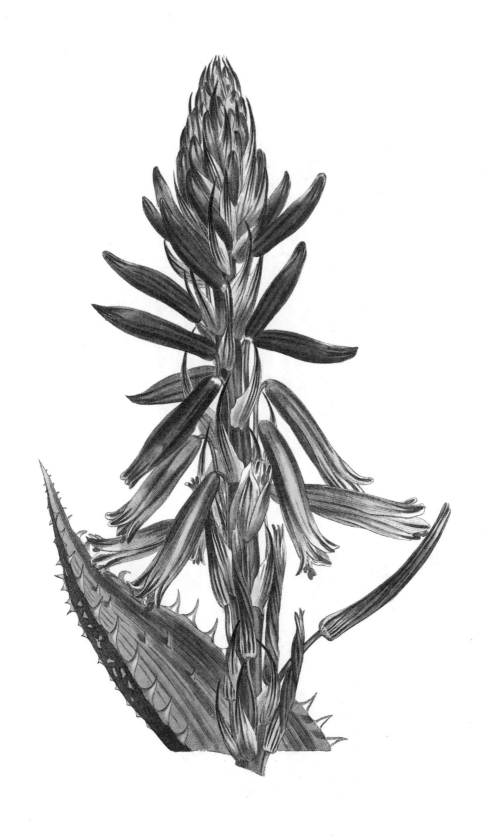

Aloe humilis — same as aloe africana — belongs to the family of Cape aloe (aloe capensis); it is at home in South Africa and Namibia. Originally it was found in the region of the Cape of Good Hope. This aloe variety is a traditional inhabitant of our botanical gardens. The curative properties develop in the leaves. They grow to about two feet. Botanists also know this aloe by the name of »soft-spined aloe«; the spines appear at the rims of the leaves.

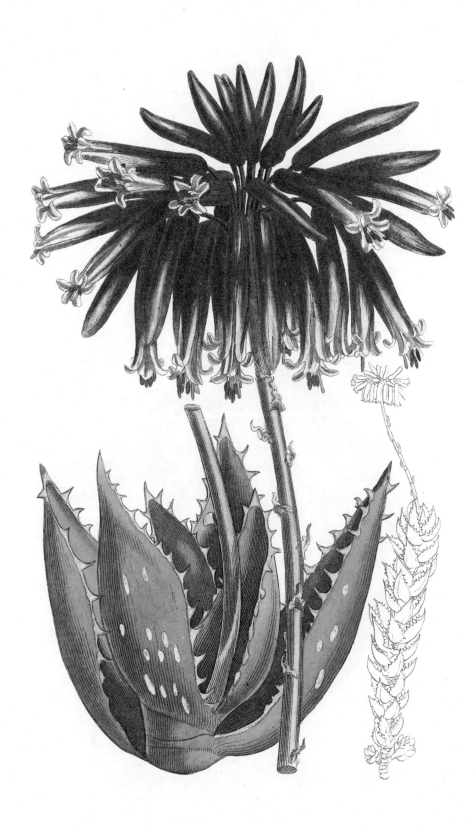

Aloe mitraeformis has its name from the shape of its leaves. If you imagine the plant upside down, the shape of a medieval mitre, i.e. the cap of a bishop or pope, appears. Among the family of the so-called mitre-aloe plants, the one depicted here is the smallest, but the one with the greatest effect of its curative substances. The mitre aloe likewise originated in the region of the Cape of Good Hope, but now it can be found in other regions as well, even in Israel and Jordan.

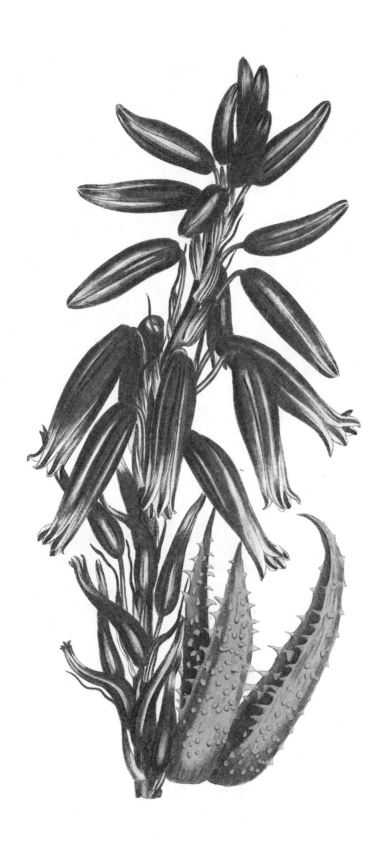

»Aloe humilis incarva« is a plant with narrow leaves coming from South Africa. It blooms profusely in many different colors, so that the sight of it pleases the eye, whether it be in the open country or in a greenhouse. The short and fleshy leaves with spines contain a lot of juice, which in popular medicine is used for the treatment of wounds and is now taking its place in scientific medical practice.

The plant shown here has been grown from seed in Kensington (England).

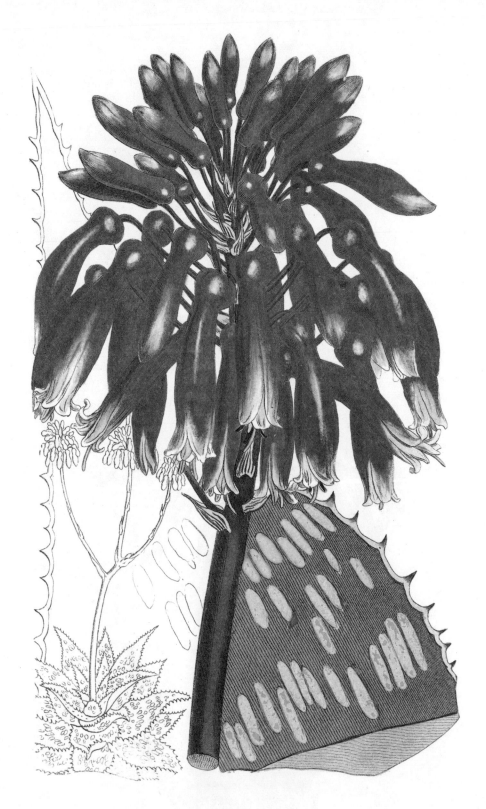

Aloe Saponaria

When the well-known botanist and explorer Miller, after whom our familiar »aloe ferox Miller« is named, traveled through the region along the Cape of Good Hope in South Africa, he made an interesting discovery: he met natives that were distinguished by an especially beautiful, smooth and shiny skin and a clear complexion. Even members of the older generation of the tribe had youthful skin and a striking appearance. Miller watched their life style and noted that these Africans pressed a white juice from the dark green leaves of a certain large aloe variety; this juice, which looks like liquid soap, they used for washing. The curative substances contained in this juice not only cleanse the pores, but have a contracting effect and offer protection from ultra-violet rays; thus they prevent the formation of wrinkles in a natural way. In this manner nature has provided an instant, liquid medicinal soap with which up to now only a handful of initiated people have been familiar.

Since its discovery by Europeans this aloe has been called aloe saponaria, i.e. soap aloe. Besides Africa it also grows in other regions with a suitable climate, such as the U.S.A. and Mexico. Other names are »Carolina aloe« and »American aloe«. Same as most other aloes, it blooms profusely in August and September. The high crown of blooms is bright red and shines like a signal from a distance.

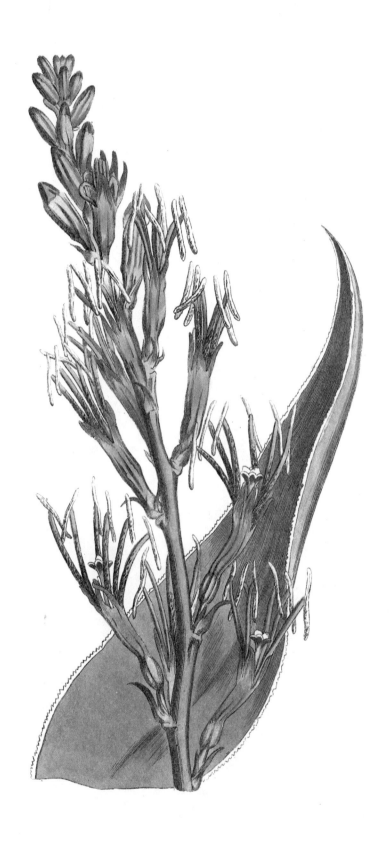

AGAVA VIRGINICA, among the most beautiful and medically potent from the family of agava americana, comes from Virginia, North and South Carolina in the U.S.A. There it was first discovered by the botanist John Cree in 1765.

The agave is known in different variations of blooms and leaves. It blooms in August and September. This variety is also called spike-flowered agave. Every plant has many blossoms. The stem of this variety grows to a height of four or five feet.

Medicaments are produced from both its blossoms (for stomach and digestion) and leaves, in which under certain circumstances biogenic stimulators develop.

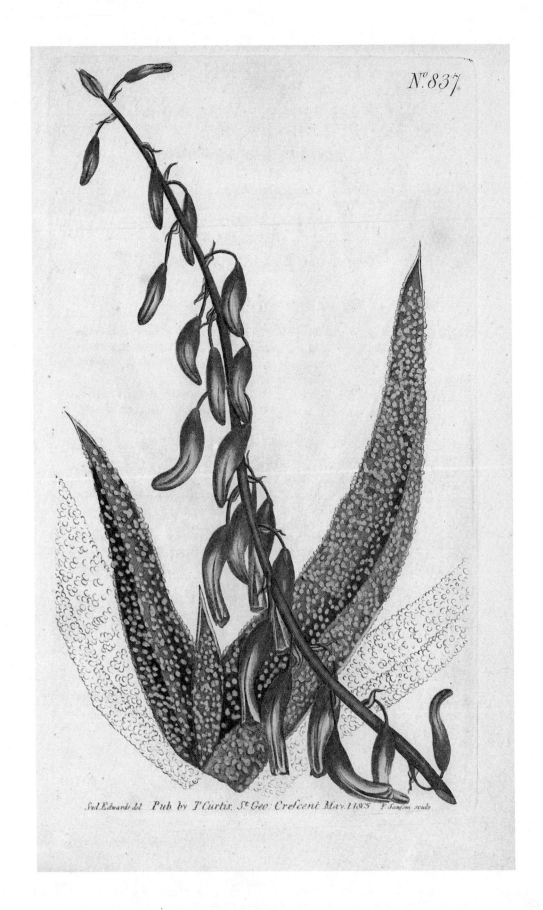

Aloe verrucosa

The striking feature of this aloe variety is its warty, sturdy leaves which contain a lot of juice. Therefore this aloe is a peculiar specialty from the Cape region. This curative plant can be found in European greenhouses. It was first cultivated by the English botanist Miller in 1731.

INFORMATION FOR THOSE SUFFERING FROM ALLERGIES

Patients highly allergic to vegetable substances are advised to reduce the recommended doses of aloe extract to no more than two injections a week of 1 ml each.

In case of allergies the doctor is to be consulted.

Research is being conducted to develop an aloe extract of a special potency for allergy patients, which has a desensitizing effect. A bio-stimulated aloe potency of this kind would considerably ameliorate the situation of allergy patients because of the invigoration of the immune defenses through the aloe healing system.

BIBLIOGRAPHY

Prof. Max Brandt, M.D., Berlin (West):
Reports of the Institute for Eastern Europe at the Free University of Berlin, issue 29, and series 18, issue 1 from August 1, 1960:
»Wege und Umwege der Sowjetmedizin« (»Ways and Detours of Soviet Medicine«)

Prof. Dr. Alfred Brauchle, **»Das große Buch der Naturheilkunde«** (»The Complete Book of Naturopathy«), Prisma Publishing House, Gütersloh, 1977

Theodor Burang **»Tibetische Heilkunde«** (»Tibetan Medicine«), Origo Publishing House, Zurich, 1974

J. F. Dastur **»Ayurvedische Medizin«** (»Ayurvedic Medicine«), published by D. B. Taraporevala Sons & Co., Bombay, India, 1978

Ming Wong **»Handbuch der Chinesischen Pflanzenheilkunde«** (»Handbook of Chinese Phytotherapy«), Publishing House Hermann Bauer, Freiburg, 1978

Dr. N. L. Arjajew **»Einfluß der Gewebetherapie auf das Zentralnervensystem«** (»Influence of Tissue Therapy on the Central Nervous System«): Filatow Institute for Ophthalmology and Tissue Therapy, Odessa

Dr. N. A. Putschkowkaja, Prof. S. R. Mutschnik, Dr. S. N. Gontscharenko **»Gewebetherapie kardiovaskulärer Erkrankungen bei Personen in vorgeschrittenem und hohem Lebensalter«** (»Tissue Therapy of Cardiovascular Diseases at an Advanced and High Age«), Odessa

Prof. Dr. Mutschnik, Dr. Solovieva **»Gewebetherapie nach der Methode Filatow«** (»Tissue Therapy according to Filatow«), Odessa

Alexander Popowski **»Auf der Grenze zwischen Leben und Tod«** (»On the Border between Life and Death«), Publishing House Kultur und Fortschritt, Berlin, 1951

Government Bulletin of the Indian state of Tamil Nadu, Madras: **»St. Thomas in Madras«**, 1976

Pschyrembel **»Klinisches Wörterbuch«** (»Clinical Dictionary«), published by de Gruyter, Berlin and New York

Welt am Sonntag, issues 49 from Dec. 2, 1984, and 24 from June 18, 1985

A. D. Turowa, E. N. Saposchnikowa **»Heilpflanzen der UdSSR«** (»Medicinal Herbs of the USSR«), Publishing House Medizin, Moscow, 1983

Deutsches Homöopathisches Arzneibuch (German Homeopathic Pharmacopoeia) Publishing House Deutscher Apotheker, Stuttgart, official edition

Dr. Christian Ullmann **»Homöopathie und Wissenschaft«** (»Homeopathy and Science«), Naturheilpraxis, issue 9/1981

Dr. A. Krumm-Helier **»Magie der Duftstoffe«** (»Magic of Odorous Substances«), Publishing House Richard Schikowski, Berlin

R. A. Hoffmann **»So besiegte ich den Krebs«** (»Thus I Defeated Cancer«) Publishing House Brigitta Hoffmann, 8963 Waltenhofen